Clean, Green, and Lean

Get Rid of the Toxins That Make You Fat

DR. WALTER CRINNION

WILEY

John Wiley & Sons, Inc.

Published by John Wiley & Sons, Inc., Hoboken, New Jersey
Published simultaneously in Canada

Design by Forty-five Degree Design LLC

The information contained in this book is not intended to serve as a replacement for professional medical advice. Any use of the information in this book is at the reader's discretion. The author and the publisher specifically disclaim any and all liability arising directly or indirectly from the use or application of any information contained in this book. A health care professional should be consulted regarding your specific situation.

Designations used by companies to distinguish their products are often claimed as trademarks. In all instances where John Wiley & Sons, Inc., is aware of a claim, the product names appear in Initial Capital or ALL CAPITAL letters. Readers, however, should contact the appropriate companies for more complete information regarding trademarks and registration.

For general information about our other products and services, please contact our Customer Care Department within the United States at (800) 762–2974, outside the United States at (317) 572–3993 or fax (317) 572–4002.

Wiley also publishes its books in a variety of electronic formats. Some content that appears in print may not be available in electronic books. For more information about Wiley products, visit our web site at www.wiley.com.

Library of Congress Cataloging-in-Publication Data:

Crinnion, Walter, date.
    Clean, green, and lean : get rid of the toxins that make you fat / Walter Crinnion.
      p. cm.
    Includes bibliographical references and index.
    ISBN 978-0-470-40923-7 (cloth)
      1. Diet—Popular works. 2. Naturopathy—Popular works. I. Title.
    [DNLM: 1. Diet—methods—Popular Works. 2. Naturopathy—methods—Popular Works. 3. Overweight—etiology—Popular Works. 4. Overweight—prevention & control—Popular Works. WB 935 C931c 2010]
  RA784.C65 2010
  613.2'5—dc26

                                              2009028778

Printed in the United States of America

10 9 8 7 6 5 4 3 2 1

This book is dedicated to all who have come to me for care.

Thank you for your faith and trust, and for providing me with so many great reasons to learn more.

And to the most fantastic woman on the planet, my wife, Kelly.

Thank you for life.

CONTENTS

Foreword by Dr. Peter D'Adamo   vii

Acknowledgments   ix

Introduction: What's Clean? Why Green? How Lean?   1

PART ONE. **Understanding and Overcoming Toxins**

1   Reduce Your Toxic Burden and Be Lean for Life   19

2   The Toxin–Fat Connection   30

PART TWO. **The Clean, Green Solution**

3   A Different Kind of Diet   57

4   Out with the Bad   80

5   Supplements: Your Secret Weapons   99

6   Your Home on a Diet   118

PART THREE. **Living Clean, Green, and Lean**

7   The Clean, Green, and Lean Four-Week Plan   149

8   Clean, Green, and Lean Recipes   198

9   A Fourteen-Day Menu Plan   246

10   Moving Forward   252

Appendix: The Link between Farmed Salmon and Diabetes   259

Notes   261

Resources   273

Index   287

FOREWORD
by Dr. Peter D'Adamo

"Woe to the book you can read without constantly wondering about the author!" wrote the Romanian philosopher and essayist E. M. Cioran. I think Cioran makes a rarely recognized and unguarded point. People write books, and it is often the personality and skills of the author that make the difference between a series of accumulated platitudes and a cogent and effective call to action.

While most of the current popular books on cleansing and detoxification approach the subject from the perspective of fantasy and folklore, this book grounds itself in evidence and positions itself firmly on the side of science. Be assured that the valuable advice you'll receive here is proven, factual, and safe. You will be reading the book finally written by the man "who wrote the book" on the subject.

Having known Dr. Walter Crinnion for over three decades, I can assure you that there is no better authority in nutritional medicine on the subjects of detoxification and cleansing. Better yet, I can report that the guidance you are about to receive from this book is given in that friendly, informal style that characterizes Walter's genuine personality and temperament and that serves to make him such a popular instructor and a much sought after lecturer.

The one characteristic of Walter's that I treasure above all others is the tremendous enthusiasm he has for this work and his mission. The word *enthusiasm* comes from the Greek *en theos,* signifying "the God within." I'm sure that you will soon be wondering about this special person, whose first book is truly the result of being blessed with the ways and means to express those essential thoughts that are inside him.

A quick study of the book's beginning, middle, and end can best allow us to appreciate the sheer conceptual scale of this work. Walter begins by taking you on a trip to the invisible world of the hidden toxins that permeate our everyday lives. He uncovers the hidden threats behind pesticides, PCBs, and DDT, and describes the nine classes of toxic compounds. In short order you'll find out how to detoxify nonorganic produce and cleanse your home environment. Walter's advice is sound and practical and ranges from the latest biochemistry and genomics to something as simple as taking your shoes off before entering your home.

After identifying the problem, the second part of the book launches into the basics of naturopathic detoxification. There is an extensive discussion of the importance of cleansing the bowels—advice as valid now as when it was first offered by Hippocrates, the father of medicine, over two thousand years ago. How to block fat absorption using safe and commonly available herbal remedies, enhancing the detoxification mechanisms of the liver and the kidneys, balancing the "good" and the "bad" estrogens in the body, and some terrific supplement advice round out the second part of the book.

The final third of the book is where your clean, green, and lean program is developed. It allows you to work toward a cleaner, greener life through a guided step-by-step approach. You'll begin by purging and reorganizing your food pantry. Then you'll learn how to keep a daily journal and use an elimination process to help identify problematic foods. This section is capped off by a terrific recipe collection and an extensive and helpful collection of outside resources.

Over the years, I've seen Dr. Walter Crinnion give patients their lives back, often as the happy ending to an otherwise sorry tale of missed diagnoses, therapeutic dead ends, and thousands of wasted dollars. It is my great honor and pleasure to introduce you to his first book.

Dr. Peter D'Adamo, a second-generation naturopathic physician, is the author of the *New York Times* bestseller *Eat Right 4 Your Type*. His book is now in its fourteenth printing in hardback and has been translated into forty other languages. He has an international following and conducts biannual conferences for those interested in the interface between diet, health, and human individuality.

ACKNOWLEDGMENTS

This book has been in the making for the last thirty years, since I first entered naturopathic medical school. I owe a debt of thanks to my teachers and mentors, Dr. John Bastyr, Dr. Joe Pizzorno, and Dr. Bill Mitchell being chief among them. My good friends and colleagues Dr. Davis Lamson, Dr. Peter D'Adamo, and Dr. Soram Khalsa have continued to inspire and encourage me along my path and have been wonderful companions.

A huge debt of thanks is due to all of my patients who have come to me for care and have taught me so much in the process. It has been a great path of partnership and co-learning, and thankfully tremendous healing for so many of them.

To my great joy, my path has led me to my soul mate, Dr. Kelly Crinnion, who has done more for my life than can be put into words. She has taken life from existence to *life*, a daily joyful existence. Our co-creative power has been phenomenal and is hugely responsible for this book coming to fruition along with our beautiful daughter, Kate. Kelly has been a fantastic source of support and is responsible for all of the wonderful recipes in this book, and as you can tell, she is also a fantastic cook. I am indeed the luckiest man in the world.

I also need to thank my fantastic agent, Janis Vallely, for working her magic to make this book happen, and to Tom Miller at John Wiley & Sons, who recognized the potential power of this information. And finally, to Doug Wagner and Toni Robino of With Flying

Colours, who provided the greatest support an author could have. They uncorked the bottle and helped my words flow smoothly onto the pages like fine wine.

To all of you, I owe my deepest thanks for your help on this delightful journey.

What's Clean? Why Green? How Lean?

How would you like to lose weight without starvation diets, count-ing calories, and complicated meal plans? With *Clean, Green, and Lean* you can—and you don't even have to exercise, although it's best if you do, of course. As an environmental medicine physician, I know that losing weight and staying healthy has more to do with getting rid of toxins in your diet, in your body, and in your environment than with following the latest diet fad. Clean up your diet, clean out your body, and clean out your house, and your extra pounds will melt away along with the toxins you eliminate. And by the way, so will most, if not all, of your health problems, including fatigue, aches and pains, allergies, depression, and other mysterious and nagging symptoms your doctor can't cure.

But there's more to this than how great you'll look and feel. Sure, you'll lose weight without being hungry or increasing the amount of exercise you do. Sure, you'll be healthier, slimmer, and more ener-getic than you've been in years. But you'll also be helping to save the planet. If you're cleaner and greener, the world will be cleaner and greener.

1

In the early 1970s, I was a premed student at the University of San Francisco. I'd wanted to be a physician ever since I was very young, and while I wasn't sure what kind of doctor I wanted to be, I knew I wanted to help people to heal. During that time, I was introduced to a woman in her seventies named Grace Bliss (how's that for a wonderful name?) who had been a big believer in health foods and natural healing since the 1940s. Because of her influence, I began to change my diet and started colon cleansing programs to reduce the amount of toxins stored in my body. When I simply took refined sugar out of my diet, I was rewarded with two extra hours of energy every day. After beginning to see the power of natural foods in my life, I wanted to learn more about how to help others heal with them. I just wasn't sure how.

Several years and another college later, I was in the lunch line when fellow student Judy Coad handed me a catalog for the National College of Naturopathic Medicine, in Portland, Oregon. Judy was trained in foot reflexology, and I'd already seen how well that worked for me when I had a horrible case of allergic sinusitis. One session with Judy and my sinuses began to drain and the oppressive headache caused by those impacted sinuses finally lifted. This was the first I'd heard of naturopathic medicine, and I asked a surgeon I knew what he thought of it. He patiently reviewed the course catalog and told me he didn't even know what some of the class names meant (pharmacognosy, for example). And it was the same story everywhere—no one I asked had ever heard of naturopathic medicine. I had a mystery on my hands, and I decided to investigate. Then there would be at least *one* person on campus who knew what it was. This was one of the best decisions of my life.

What I discovered is that naturopathic medicine is a distinct medical system of health care: an art, science, and practice of diagnosing and treating people and preventing disease. Naturopathic physicians seek to restore and maintain optimal health through the use of natural remedies such as diet, nutritional supplements, physical therapy, and homeopathic remedies. Naturopathic medicine honors patients as unique human beings, enabling them to take responsibility for their own health.

Today, I'm surrounded by colleagues who, like myself, have found naturopathic medicine to be their calling, not their job. I have yet to meet a naturopathic physician who entered the field for financial stability or to achieve a respected place in society. Most of us simply feel called to help heal others and the planet through this profession.

My own path led me to become a member of the first graduating class at what's now known as Bastyr University, in Kenmore, Washington. At Bastyr I was privileged to learn from Dr. Bastyr himself, along with Dr. Joe Pizzorno (president of the university and coauthor of the *Textbook of Natural Medicine*) and Dr. Bill Mitchell. Besides learning from these gifted healers, I found myself working alongside brilliant classmates such as Peter D'Adamo. Of course, he's now Dr. Peter D'Adamo, author of *Eat Right 4 Your Type*. Through his book and seminars, Dr. D'Adamo has helped thousands of people enjoy better health.

Upon graduation I began my general family practice, including offering natural childbirth services, and ended up focusing on food allergies and sensitivities. When my patients were willing to avoid the foods I had identified as being most likely to cause problems, the most wonderful things happened. I saw seasonal allergies, migraines, arthritis, eczema, asthma, angina, and even seizures and schizophrenia improve and in many cases disappear. While most physicians would be satisfied with finding the culprits behind the problems, I wanted to do more: I wanted to help these people get over their reactions so that they wouldn't have to keep those foods out of their diets forever.

This quest is what led me in the direction of environmental medicine. Starting with the old naturopathic idea of liver cleansing to combat food reactions, I embarked on a learning journey that included trial and error and lots of days and nights studying at the Health Science Library at the University of Washington. As I began to perform more liver cleansings, more patients began to show up at my door. They brought with them a host of symptoms and health problems that I'd never heard about in medical school, such as chemical sensitivity and fibromyalgia. I'd sit in my office and listen to people who looked just fine to me describe how they ended up with awful health problems after merely smelling a chemical that I'd smelled hundreds of times without a problem. I made a decision that no matter what the symptom looked or sounded like, I would believe what my patients told me and do my best to help them. That resolution changed my medical career.

From there I began to specialize in working with environmentally poisoned people. Soon I began to refer to my practice as the caboose on the train of health because by the time patients got to me, they had been to everybody else and had spent thousands of dollars. Another well-known naturopathic physician who had his practice in my office at the time told me, "Walter, I don't want to see any of your patients. They're all complicated cases." And it was true. I began to get patients with complex problems that seemed to defy both allopathic (standard medical) and naturopathic treatments.

Looking for the Cause: A Radical Notion?

In allopathic medicine, the focus is on treating the symptoms. If your presenting symptom is high blood pressure, you get a pill to lower it. If you have headaches or arthritis, you get pills to ease your pain. But what's causing these symptoms is rarely even considered. Naturopathic medicine fills this gap. Our medicine is based on a set of principles that includes *Tolle causum*, or treat the cause. Is the high blood pressure caused by a deficiency of blood pressure medication in the blood? Are headaches caused by an aspirin deficiency? Of course not. If we can identify the cause of the problems and use natural means to deal with it, we can effect a *real* cure—a cure not only for the symptoms at hand but also for further symptoms. This is one reason that licensed naturopathic physicians are so good at treating chronic illnesses that have been difficult for the allopathic world to treat successfully.

When looking at a patient, most naturopathic and naturally minded physicians ask themselves what natural substance or technique the patient needs to make him or her better. Is it a vitamin or mineral deficiency? Is there an herb that works especially well for the problem? Does he or she need a spinal adjustment, acupuncture, or a homeopathic remedy? And for the most part, these natural supplements and treatments work exceptionally well. My family and I have used them for some time and can attest to their benefits. But sometimes patients are ill not because they're deficient in something but because they have too much toxicity. And this has led to a radical new way to view natural medicine, one in which the question is what do we need to take away rather than what do we need to add. This book will show you what you need to take away—besides the weight.

Every one of us is living in a toxic world. We're born with a body burden of chemicals we inherit while still in the womb because chemicals in our mother's body cross the placenta into ours. Just by living an ordinary life from that point on we're accumulating additional traces every day, and over the years it adds up to frightening levels. We breathe in toxins when we walk down the soap aisle at the grocery store and when we do our laundry with scented detergent and fabric softener. We absorb toxins from carpeting, paint, and cabinets in our homes and workplaces and from meals microwaved in plastic. In other words, just by living in this day and age, we silently and without doing anything alarming build up a toxic load. Moving through our bloodstream along with nutrients, oxygen, and other essentials that our body needs is a host of chemicals—chemicals that were manufactured to help us live a better life but weren't intended to be inside of us. A lab could have a field day listing all of the toxins floating around in our blood and urine.

Most of these chemicals have been studied and shown to be toxic to animals and humans. But very few of us have enough of any one of them for toxicologists to classify us as poisoned. That typically requires some sort of accidental industrial overload. But these chemicals are still toxins, and when they're combined, they form an overwhelming load in our bodies. What's shocking to me is that the scientists and government officials charged with oversight in this area are so slow to understand this fact. The method of proof that worked so well to identify the bacteria or virus responsible for each of the major infectious diseases just doesn't work when we're dealing with this toxic deluge. It's like arguing about which drop of rain made the rain barrel overflow.

Despite the fact that every high school chemistry student learns this basic science of combined effects, it took the National Research Council (NRC) until this year to release a report addressing chemicals' cumulative impact. Naturopathic physicians have known for decades that the federal pollution standard seriously underestimates the collective effects of chemicals. The Environmental Protection Agency (EPA) and the Food and Drug Administration (FDA) usually test the impact of chemicals individually. The NRC is now saying, finally, that this approach could underestimate the health impact of being exposed to a variety of chemicals simultaneously. The "straw that broke the camel's back" is a good analogy for what can happen when individual toxins build up in our bodies and reach critical mass. As individual compounds, toxins cause adverse health effects, and, not surprisingly, when combined these poisons make us sick. They make us tired. And they make us fat.

Americans' average toxic burden is higher than it's ever been. At the same time, our rate of obesity is off the charts. Coincidence? I don't think so. In fact, several scientific studies that I cite in this book show a strong correlation between levels of toxic burden and both higher body weight and the risk of diabetes. So, from a toxicity point of view, it's not surprising that diabetes and being overweight go hand in hand.

It's also true that we all carry a toxic burden but not all of us are fat. Some of us may be better at fighting back. We can't escape toxin exposure altogether, but we can cut it way back. We can protect ourselves from what we can't avoid and get rid of a large portion of the toxins our bodies have stored up. And we can do this without extreme measures. All it takes are some basic lifestyle adjustments and some all-natural supplements to our diets. All in all, the strategy I propose in this book is a simple one. These are the goals:

- Stop new toxins from coming *into* the body.
- Get accumulated toxins *out* of the body.

The ways to accomplish these goals are simple, too:

- Clean up your diet.
- Clean up your home environment.
- Use toxin-fighting supplements.
- Improve elimination.

Believe it—we *can* heal.

As I've mentioned, by eliminating reactive foods from their diets— the top three being wheat, sugar, and dairy—my patients often found great relief from their problems. But what was causing them to react to these foods in the first place? As it turned out, being toxically burdened was a major factor (though not the sole cause), and one that could be remedied by reducing toxins and making sure they wouldn't build up again. I was truly amazed at the breadth of medical problems that were helped by cleansing the body the way I'm going to show you in this book. It's not simply about detoxing, which amounts to turning toxic compounds in your body into something nontoxic. It's about going a step further and getting rid of these compounds entirely.

To achieve this, you'll have to buy organic versions of certain foods, be careful about which fish you eat, increase the amount of a few key foods in your diet, and use certain all-natural supplements that help your body get rid of fat. You'll have to put your home on a diet, too, cleaning out the many common household products that harbor toxic components and replacing them with alternatives that are gentler on both your body and the environment.

In the first part of the book, you'll learn all about toxins and why they're making your otherwise healthy life miserable. In part two, I'll explain what you can do to win the war on toxins and reap the benefits of losing weight and getting healthier. Know right away that this is a relatively easy process. I've created a four-week plan for you that tells you exactly what you need to do. So relax, take a deep breath, and prepare to see the fat begin to melt away. Forget you ever heard the phrase "calories in, calories out." Those days are over. The operative phrase for the new era of your life is "toxins out, pounds off."

We all know the problem with calories in, calories out diets: They don't work, at least not for many people. Even people with willpower fail. Even gym rats keep putting on the pounds. They cut fat, give up carbs, or weigh every serving of food, or they exercise with a stopwatch for interval training or wear a pedometer to make sure they get their 10,000 steps—and they still can't get rid of the excess weight. Or, even worse, they lose weight but yo-yo right back in six months, which is very hard on the internal organs. Despite their best efforts, most people fail when it comes to losing weight and keeping it off. That's because they've missed the most important variable: toxins. Stop letting them into your body, and get rid of what's already stockpiled there. Then your body will be free to release the fat it has been holding on to to protect itself, and your metabolism will pick up the pace.

Don't get me wrong—you're not off the hook when it comes to exercising. It's one of my main recommendations for patients and has far-reaching benefits for your health. Our bodies were designed to be active and fit—that's what makes them work and feel best. I'm all for healthy food choices and sensible portions, too. Exercise and eat well, and you'll be healthier all around. You'll also lose weight faster. But the main purpose of this book is for you to discover, firsthand, that it's simple, relatively easy, and very rewarding to live a clean, green, and lean lifestyle.

It Really Works!

After guiding patients through my cleansing program for a number of years, I began to wonder whether I was selectively remembering only the patients it had worked for and was blocking out the memory of those who hadn't had such great results. Was I in a version of *The Emperor's New Clothes* and not aware of it? We all have the ability to see the world around us in the way we want to see it and in a way that's favorable to us. Is that what I was doing, or was this method of healing indeed as effective as I thought it was? To find out, I did a study of all of the patients who'd gone through my cleansing program in the previous five years. This entailed sending out questionnaires (allowing the patients to remain anonymous) about the state of their health before and after cleansing. I entered into this study with some fears—what if I really wasn't helping people?—but didn't let them stop me. In retrospect, I realize what a rare action this was to take. I can think of only one other physician, Dr. Dean Ornish, president and founder of the nonprofit Preventive Medicine Research Institute in Sausalito, California, and clinical professor of medicine at the University of California, San Francisco, who studied his patients to see whether what he was doing was actually working. What my staff and I found from the study astounded all of us: we were helping people more than we could have imagined.

We had asked people to list their main health complaints (the ones that bothered them the most and prompted them to do the cleansing work) and to grade the improvements that followed cleansing. I tabulated the results in the chart on page 9, and they were published in the *Journal of Naturopathic Medicine*.

RESULTS OF FIFTEEN OR MORE SESSIONS OF TISSUE CLEANSING AND RESTORATION PROGRAM

Complaints	Worse	No Change	Slight Change	Moderate/ Good	Great	Total
MCS	0	2	1	8	13	24
Autoimmune	0	0	0	4	12	16
Neurologic	0	3	2	4	6	15
Fatigue	0	1	0	6	7	14
Cancer	0	2	0	2	4	8
Allergies	0	0	1	5	1	7
General cleansing	0	0	2	5	0	7
Musculoskeletal	0	0	2	2	1	5
Dermatological	0	0	0	3	1	4
Respiratory	0	0	0	0	3	3
GI/liver	0	0	0	1	2	3
General debility	0	1	1	0	1	3
HIV/AIDS	0	0	1	1	0	2
Addictions	0	0	0	0	1	1
Totals	0	9	10	41	52	112
Percent	0	8	9	36.60	46.40	100

You can see from the table that no one's condition worsened after the treatment, and the vast majority—83 percent—of the people who'd done the cleansing work by this point reported good to great improvement. Included in this are sixteen patients whose prime complaint was some form of autoimmunity, a condition in which the immune system goes haywire and attacks body tissues. Their diagnoses included Hashimoto's thyroiditis, rheumatoid arthritis, psoriatic arthritis, multiple sclerosis, scleroderma, Sjögren's syndrome, silicone-related connective tissue disorder, and lupus. All of these sixteen patients rated their improvement as good or great, with 75 percent of them reporting great improvement.

According to the medical establishment, there's no cure for autoimmune illnesses—there are only medications to help relieve the symptoms. These illnesses are thought of as being chronic, progressive problems. They don't go away; rather, they continue to get worse over time. Yet these sixteen people experienced miraculous (and I don't use that word lightly) turnarounds. Though I'd never learned in medical school that toxic burden causes autoimmune illnesses, I don't believe these results were a coincidence.

That twenty-one of the twenty-four patients with multiple chemical sensitivity (MCS) experienced good to great improvement wasn't a surprise at all, as MCS is clearly associated with chemical exposures. What was a surprise was how consistently these people were able to regain their health. If you go to support groups for people with chemical sensitivity, you'll hear only the horror stories about how it continues to progress and get worse. But I have patients who went through my cleansing program and no longer consider themselves chemically sensitive.

The components of my cleansing protocol are nothing new—sauna, hydrotherapy, and colonic irrigations—but apparently the order and frequency are. My protocol has provided great healing for a wide variety of the most common health problems of our times.

Discovering the Link among Green, Clean, and Lean

Another major lesson I learned from my patients was not to overtreat them. I realized I didn't need to give them supplementation or other forms of treatment for their individual health problems. I already had them on plenty of supplements for basic support of the body's biochemistry, and I didn't want them to take more. I found that as they reduced their toxic loads, their other health problems began to get better on their own. This is one of the other great principles of naturopathic medicine: *vis medicatrix naturae*, or "the healing power of nature," which encompasses the body's ability to heal itself.

I discovered that I didn't need to give immune-support nutrients to people with chronic viral infections or chronic fatigue. I just needed to cleanse them. When their toxic levels dropped, their white blood cells began to attack the viruses just as they're supposed to. I didn't have to give a lot of adrenal support to people with chronic adrenal insufficiency, because their adrenal glands would also begin to heal. When patients reduced their toxic burdens, all of their organs started to work much better. They typically experienced an increase in energy and mental clarity and would often tell me that they felt twenty years younger. It was like being in a sneaker commercial—after cleansing, my patients were able to run faster and jump higher. Talk about a fountain of youth. And I also had the delightful fortune to start hearing my patients say things like, "Doc, I haven't changed my diet at all, but since cleansing it's like the pounds are falling off all by themselves." They weren't on a calorie-counting diet, they hadn't started an intense exercise program—they were just cleaner! And the cleaner and greener they got, the leaner they got. It seemed that I had a front-row seat for the unfolding of daily miracles. It wasn't until twenty years after I started cleansing work with patients that I discovered why all this was happening.

Mitochondria are inside every cell in every living thing on the planet, including humans. They provide power for cells by creating energy from fats and sugars, driving the metabolism and the whole body. When toxins damage these cellular power plants, they can't work effectively or efficiently—sluggish mitochondria make for a sluggish metabolism. In turn, the fats and sugars that they aren't burning for fuel pile up all over the body in the form of extra pounds. Further, when ailing mitochondria don't provide your cells with the energy they need, you're not going to have the energy you need. This is a frequent yet largely unknown cause of the fatigue and exhaustion so common in today's world.

With this valuable new knowledge in hand, I wanted to expand my circle of influence. Teaching in my office with limited seating space would allow a limited number of people to take advantage of what I had to offer, but if I could teach others about the field of environmental medicine, many more people could be helped. So I began to channel much of my energy into teaching naturopathic, allopathic, and chiropractic physicians about this field: how to spot the classic presentation of environmental toxic overload, how to test for it, and how to treat it. As a result, I've shared my information with many wonderful and dedicated professionals, some of whom have really taken it to heart and have become teachers to me.

But I also wanted to get this lifesaving information to the people in need. After all, it's your health that's being affected. You're the one who's toxic. Another principle of naturopathic medicine is *docere*, or doctor as teacher, and I've always tried to make medical information understandable to my patients. I make sure they have copies of all of their lab work and understand what the test results mean. I believe that the more they understand what's going on in their bodies and what the process of healing entails, the more empowered they will be to make it all happen. I don't speak in Latin, I don't wear a white coat, and you don't have to call me Doctor. But I do know what's going on physically in my patients, and they need to know it, too. They're the ones who will heal themselves—I just get to assist in the process. In the same way, I'll assist you in this book.

As we clear from our bodies the chemicals that are keeping us from being the vibrant people we're meant to be, we can begin to step into our true potential. As each person becomes more whole, I believe, the planet as a whole becomes more whole. And this also brings forth a less toxic legacy for our children's children. The Iroquois tribe used to make decisions by asking what the impact would be seven generations down from themselves. One wonders whether, if the captains of industry had asked the same question, we'd be in the toxic soup we're now in.

We may not be captains of industry, but we're all decision makers. Every day with our food purchases, we make decisions that influence how many pesticides are sprayed around the globe. We decide how many hydrocarbons are emitted into the air by the way we commute. We decide how many solvents and plastics will be in our children's bodies with the purchases we make and how we cook our food. If we all choose to start living less toxic lives, the entire planet will benefit. You really do have the power to make a profound difference, for yourself, your family, and the rest of the world.

As I continued to hear my patients' stories, I was struck by how normal all of their lives were. I'd thought that because I was in Seattle, I'd end up treating a lot of people who worked around toxic compounds in the aerospace industry. In fact, I had very few toxic patients who worked in any kind of toxic environment. The vast majority of my patients were housewives or office workers—not what you'd expect to be highly toxic professions. And almost none of them had had toxic episodes, where they were exposed to levels of a compound that would make a toxicologist sit up and pay attention. No, most of these patients became ill slowly, with the symptoms creeping up on them and then getting worse just a little at a time—the same way that we accumulate toxins, just a little at a time. These patients came in with the same chronic complaints that are presented to health professionals all over the country. They came in with fatigue, depression, headaches, asthma, allergies, arthritis, and a host of other common problems, including three of the biggies—heart disease, cancer, and parkinsonism. They'd simply been going about their lives as we all do, and at some point they had experienced one exposure too many. Many of them weren't even aware of what that exposure was because it was so ordinary. All they knew was that they'd begun to lose their health. Others could identify the exposure that had kicked them over the edge and wanted to blame it for all of their problems. But for every one of them, the cause was actually the same: the total load of toxins had become too great for their bodies to handle.

I was shocked by the realization that normal, everyday exposure is what made my patients ill, and I wanted to avoid following any of them on the paths they'd gone down. Ever hear about the miners of old taking a canary into the coal mine so that when the canary died, they'd know it was time to leave? Well, all of my toxic patients became my personal canaries. I knew I really wasn't much different from any of them. And if daily exposure to toxins made them ill, it could certainly do the same to me. I also realized that there was no way to tell how close I was to experiencing one exposure too many. So I began to implement in my own life all of the things I told my patients to do in theirs. The carpet came out of my house. The furnace filters were upgraded and changed regularly. My backyard organic garden grew every year, and we bought organic food at our local co-op.

More than twenty years have passed since I began my work in environmental medicine, and I still live this way. When my wife and I decided to conceive, we tested her to find out what her toxic burden was, and she worked for over a year to reduce it before she became pregnant. We continue to buy organic foods and have been thrilled that our local grocery store now has so much to choose from. Our pantry and our home in general are chemical-free zones. I want our daughter's body to have fewer toxins than ours, not more. And I want my grandchildren to have even fewer. I want to turn this process around so that the world becomes less toxic, not more. If you'd like the same and are willing to work at it, I'll show you how you can achieve it. The world will be that much better for your efforts.

One of the biggest changes my patients consistently report is how much more tuned in to life they become once they start on the path mapped out in this book. Before they began cleansing and learning about healthy, safe choices, they were relatively unconscious of what they put into their bodies and how their diet made them feel. When they were hungry, they'd eat whatever looked or smelled good and was most convenient. When I have patients keep track of what they eat with a diet diary for a few days, they invariably come back and say, "This isn't a typical diet for me—I really eat much better than this." But the diet diary doesn't lie. It shows how they're really eating, not how they think they're eating.

Most people just don't pay attention to what they eat, but once they start cleansing, they become more aware of how their bodies feel after eating certain foods and being around certain chemicals. They also start to note how they feel when they're with certain people or watch certain TV shows or listen to certain music. They start to recognize what nurtures them and works for them and what doesn't. Then they start to let go of the people, places, and things that aren't serving their best interests. They begin to let go of emotional, energetic. and spiritual toxins along with the physical toxins. Their feelings had always been there to tell them what worked for them and what didn't—they just weren't paying attention to them. But through following my program, they begin to be aware. And this awareness may be the biggest gift my program can bring you. It can help you be more fully present in the moment and consciously choose that which is the most nurturing and life-giving for you. And in the process, you just might be helping to save the world.

Assess Your Toxic Burden and Your Health

Every journey obviously needs a starting place, but not just because it's a place to start. It's also a gauge for measuring how far you've gone, which in turn tells you how close you are to your next stop. It's important to keep things in perspective—not to become fixated on the destination or any other point. Keep in mind that this is a process—enjoy the whole trip. That said, what are your physical, mental, emotional, and spiritual starting points? You need to take stock of your current situation so that you can note all of the improvements and changes you're going to make (and so you can give yourself a huge pat on the back for each one).

Let's start with your physical health. Here is a list of the most common symptoms of toxicity and the most common health problems associated with toxins. Review the list and on a scale of 1 to 10, with 10 being the most troubling, give a score to all that apply to you.

RATE YOUR PHYSICAL TOXIC SYMPTOMS

Symptom or Health Problem	How It Rates Now (1–10)
Fatigue	
Depression	
Brain fog	
Balance problems	
Poor memory	
Headaches	
Tremors	
Allergies	
Asthma	
Chemical sensitivity	
Diabetes	
Fibromyalgia	
Autoimmunity (rheumatoid arthritis, lupus, etc.)	
Infertility	
Chronic infections	
Bone marrow problems	
Parkinsonism	
Other	
Other	
Other	

PART ONE

Understanding and Overcoming Toxins

CHAPTER 1

Reduce Your Toxic Burden and Be Lean for Life

Jackie, a thirty-eight-year-old math teacher, had strong willpower, exercised three times a week, and tried to make healthy food choices, but her excess fat stubbornly held on. At 5 feet 3 inches tall and 183 pounds, she knew she should go to the gym more often, but she was so tired after school every day that nothing could compete with her living room sofa. She might have felt more motivated to exercise if she'd been able to keep off the weight the last time she lost it, but no matter what she did, she always gained back the extra pounds and then some. As it is for millions of people worldwide, yo-yo dieting was a way of life for Jackie.

People think obesity is caused by overeating and lack of exercise, but there's more to this epidemic than meets the eye. Jackie had been blaming her fat for her fatigue, but the fatigue and the fat were caused by the same culprits: environmental toxins in her body. I assured her that if she reduced her load of toxins, she would have more energy and fewer pounds of fat.

There's no delicate way of putting it, so we may as well face the plain, hard fact: we're all toxic. And that's one of the biggest reasons that so many people are overweight. While not everyone with a heavy toxic burden is fat—and not everyone who's fat has a heavy toxic burden—all of my overweight patients who rid themselves of toxins automatically lose weight. Unfortunately, it doesn't work the other way around. Getting rid of the fat doesn't get rid of the toxins. They're reabsorbed by your body, and new fat immediately starts to collect around them. That's why losing weight without detoxing is the first step in gaining weight. It's why millions of people worldwide are fighting a losing battle. To win, you need to fight the toxins. And when you do, you also get rid of the fat and all of the other health problems associated with cells damaged by those toxins, including type 2 (adult-onset) diabetes and chronic viral infections. As your toxic levels go down, you'll lose excess weight naturally, and without a lot of struggle.

Toxins Make and Keep You Fat

Now you know why, despite their best efforts, most people fail when it comes to losing weight. Like Jackie, they don't know that they're fighting the wrong battle. When you fight the real enemy—toxins—you win the battle of the bulge once and for all.

If you've been beating yourself up for not being able to lose weight and keep it off, it's time to give yourself a break and place the blame where it rightfully belongs. Like most people who are overweight, you've been at an unfair disadvantage without knowing it. The more toxins your body is storing, the more fat you're likely to accumulate and retain. It's no coincidence that American obesity levels are rising side by side with environmental toxin levels. In 1990, less than 10 percent of the population in ten states was obese, and not a single state had an obesity rate higher than 14 percent, according to the Centers for Disease Control and Prevention. But by 2006—just sixteen years later—only four states had obesity rates under 20 percent. Twenty-two states had topped 25 percent, and two (Mississippi and West Virginia) had ballooned past the 30 percent mark.

All in all, 60 million Americans are obese, and more than 9 million of them are six to nineteen years old. Between the toxic food

> ## Are Toxins Responsible for That Big Number on Your Scale?
>
> If you're more than 10 pounds overweight and are experiencing any of the following symptoms, your toxic load is probably contributing to your weight problem.
> - Asthma and allergies
> - Cognitive problems (brain fog)
> - Depression
> - Fatigue
> - Headaches
> - Memory problems
> - Chronic pain

conveniently located at any fast-food drive-through and the toxin-laden foods that fill the shelves of most grocery stores, children have the deck stacked against them. The kids who spend more time in front of a computer, DVD player, or television screen than actively using their muscles to play and get exercise are at an even greater disadvantage. And ultimately, obesity is a problem that many people never conquer once it's taken hold.

The United Nations reported that in the year 2000, 800 million people worldwide suffered from malnutrition. That's a sobering statistic for sure. But the statistic that made my jaw drop is that 1 billion people suffered from overnutrition. And that excess food is loaded not only with calories that people don't need, but also with toxins.

The first time I met with Jackie, I knew her body was on toxic overload. In addition to the fact that she was overweight, all of Jackie's health complaints had an autoimmune component. That means that her body was mistakenly mounting an attack against its own cells and tissues in a desperate attempt to rid itself of a lifetime of accumulated poisons. When a body is functioning the way it should, only the white blood cells that can tell the difference between the body and the invading organisms enter the bloodstream. Those that can't tell the difference are eliminated. But Jackie's body wasn't eliminating all of the white cells that couldn't tell the difference, so her immune system wasn't working properly. The effects of autoimmunity don't just diminish the body's ability to fight infection—the condition also speeds up the production of antibodies, which lead the attack. Many environmental chemicals such as pesticides, solvents, and formaldehyde cause the body to produce these antibodies. When this happens, not only does the toll the toxins take make you tired and fat, but it also makes you sick—very sick.

Autoimmune illnesses include the likes of rheumatoid arthritis, lupus, and connective-tissue disorders like scleroderma and Sjögren's syndrome, all of which are quite common and strongly tied to toxic burden. In a recent study of my patients with autoimmune illnesses, every one of them who did a comprehensive cleansing program like the one outlined in this book reported good or great results.

In Jackie's case, it was clear that we had to lower her toxic burden before any weight loss or healing was possible. Those toxins were creating the vicious high-weight/low-health cycle she was caught in by damaging the mitochondria in her cells and slowing her metabolism to a snail's pace. Mitochondria are organelles—tiny structures inside each cell—that serve as the cells' power plant. They drive the metabolism by taking fats and sugars that are stored in fat tissue and turning them into fuel known as ATP (adenosine triphosphate), which provides all of the power that a body needs to be healthy.

When toxins enter the body and move throughout the tissues, they come into contact with the mitochondria and damage them. Mercury, for example, causes oxidative—or free radical—damage to the mitochondria, preventing energy production and often leading to early cell death. In one study, 48 percent of the mercury that was found inside the individual cells was found in the mitochondria themselves.

All of your body's systems—tissues, bones, muscles, brain, heart, lungs—rely on ATP fuel to function properly; every one of your body's trillions of cells depends on it. When your mitochondria are producing ATP, your body has plenty of fuel to maintain good health, and you feel vibrant and energetic. When your mitochondria are in tip-top condition, your body naturally seeks its optimal weight—and finds it—unless you consume far more calories than you need.

Is Your Excess Fat Hiding Toxins That Are Making You Sick?

If you're more than 25 pounds above your ideal weight and you're suffering from one or more of the following illnesses, your body is telling you that it's in toxic overload.

- Allergies
- Asthma
- Autoimmune disease (lupus, rheumatoid arthritis, Hashimoto's thyroiditis)
- Bone marrow cancer (lymphomas, leukemias, multiple myeloma)
- Chemical sensitivity
- Chronic fatique
- Chronic infection
- Diabetes
- Fibromyalgia
- Infertility
- Parkinsonism

The difference between optimal and minimal mitochondrial function is the difference between living life to its fullest and barely living at all. Lance Armstrong undoubtedly has great-functioning mitochondria. His body can translate a normal amount of food into enough energy to fly up the Alps and the Pyrenees Mountains. Though he starts with the same basic body, training, and diet as his competitors, he can get more rpms out of his legs than the others can. This is due to the mitochondria's ability to produce energy. When all of the mitochondria in your body are at their peak, your physical and mental potential soars. When the mitochondria fall from that peak, your metabolism slows down—which means it takes longer to burn calories—and you start putting on weight. The fats and sugars the mitochondria are supposed to burn for fuel turn into unwanted pounds. You become more and more sluggish, and your body gets fatter and fatter as it tries unsuccessfully to rev itself up. It can no longer burn fat the way it's intended to because thermogenesis—the process that burns fat to make heat and keeps your body temperature at a normal 98.6 degrees Fahrenheit—has been impaired. You may also start noticing physical, mental, and emotional limitations and eventually come down with diseases and other health problems.

Speaking of which, it turned out that Jackie was suffering from severe fibromyalgia, a debilitating disorder that causes almost constant pain. I've found the condition to be strongly associated with an overburden of environmental and emotional toxins, and the pain keeps people from being able to exercise, making it easier to gain weight and harder to lose it. On top of it all, Jackie was plagued by fatigue, another problem associated with mitochondria that aren't providing energy as they should. Anyone who has ever experienced low blood sugar knows that you become fatigued and cranky and your brain doesn't work right. That's because your mitochondria haven't had enough raw fuel to make energy. Fatigue is one of the top five complaints among people exposed to industrial chemicals, and Jackie had been so tired for so long that she'd started to think it was the normal result of a day of teaching.

The cause of all of Jackie's problems wasn't that she was lacking willpower or that she just mysteriously became ill; it was that her total toxic load was too high. The first thing she needed to do was lower her toxic burden so that her mitochondria could begin to heal. We worked toward this goal by reducing the amount of toxins she was taking in and cleansing to get rid of the toxins she already had. After just a few weeks, her cleaner body allowed her mitochondria to return to full power, resuming their vital production of ATP fuel. Her energy level improved dramatically, and her health improved across the board.

While this may sound too good to be true, it is common among people who adopt a clean, green lifestyle. If you aren't happy with the way your body looks or feels, or you're not experiencing much joy in your life, focus on healing your mitochondria. As Jackie quickly discovered, just a few easy changes can make a world of difference.

Jackie was astonished that after living with chronic fatigue, obesity, and fibromyalgia for years, it took only a few weeks for her energy to return and her weight to start dropping. It took a little longer for her pain to disappear—almost four months—but after living with it for years, she could hardly believe it was gone. For weeks, she kept thinking the pain would return, but it didn't. These are the kinds of results you can expect when you treat the cause of your health problems, including obesity.

Treating the cause means becoming educated about toxins and being vigilant about keeping as many of them out of your life as possible. My goal is to make that as simple for you as I possibly can. The first step is increasing your awareness by learning that toxins are lurking in all sorts of food and household products that you've been thinking of as safe or possibly even good for you. At least 15 trillion pounds of chemicals are manufactured or imported in the United States every year, and, as a result, more than 400 chemical contaminants have been found in human fat. Everybody has them. They're the "weight" we all carry around. You may not have all 400-plus contaminants that can be reliably identified and measured, but you can bet you have scores of them as well as dozens of others that we don't have tests for yet. And you have plenty of company. Silicon Valley assembly-line workers and organic farmers, great-grandmothers and newborn babies, couch potatoes and health nuts all have dozens of toxins stored in their bodies. No one's immune.

With hundreds of research reports that explain our toxic burden in painful detail, the question is no longer whether we have toxins in our bodies but how many and which ones. As with so many of the maladies afflicting people today, if you're overweight and suffering brain fog or chronic fatigue, you need to assess your toxic burden and take measures to lower it.

Weight Loss: The Double-Edged Sword

Jackie said she almost reached her goal weight of 135 pounds several times, but each time she became so worn out that she'd get sick and stop exercising. Then she'd start eating comfort foods, and in no time she'd put the pounds back on. What she didn't realize was that she felt worn out and got sick because she was losing weight faster than her body could rid itself of the toxins that had been stored in her fat. In fact, there was a higher percentage of toxins in her bloodstream now that she was dropping the pounds.

Yes, it's a strange situation. Though fat-stored toxins are a factor in becoming overweight, you don't lose the toxins just by losing the weight. When the stored fat is mobilized into your bloodstream, fat-soluble toxins—toxins that dissolve in fat and take up residence there—are also released. This breakdown of fat, known as lipolysis, takes place daily—especially at night, when your body goes hours without eating. When you're dieting, exercising, or experiencing high stress, your lipolysis rate increases, and that means a higher than normal amount of persistent poisons is swimming in your bloodstream along with the fats.

The owner of several Curves franchises in the Southeast recently told me he's seen many middle-aged women work out for a couple of months but begin to feel ill when they start losing weight, which robs them of their motivation to keep working out. Fatigue takes hold, and just like Jackie, they often have other classic toxic symptoms such as headache and a flulike feeling. Mood swings can also result from the higher toxic presence. The only solution: breaking the toxin recirculation cycle.

You can burn the fat for fuel in your cells, but you can't burn the fat-soluble toxins. And they aren't automatically eliminated. Although your kidneys and bowels eliminate waste, they're designed to recycle fats and oils because they're valuable nutrients needed for survival. Yes, good fats are a necessary part of physical and mental health, but your body can't tell the difference between fat and fat-soluble toxins. Your body just knows that fats are valuable and wants to hold on to them. So when a pesticide tries to leave your body by way of one of the standard routes, the recycling system designed for your survival grabs the fat-soluble toxins and puts them back into circulation. That's why these pesticides are called persistent organic pollutants (POPs)—they persist in your body. When researchers measured levels of chlorinated pesticides in adults who lost weight through either a calorie-restricted diet or stomach-stapling surgery, they found that the more weight the people in the study lost, the higher the pesticide levels in their bodies became. Those who completed the three-month calorie-restriction program lost an average of 12 percent of their total body weight, and the level of pesticides in their blood increased by 24 percent. The circulating toxin level rose twice as much as the rate of weight loss. Pesticide levels also rose in the people who had the stapling procedure. Three months after surgery, they'd lost an average of 21 percent of their weight, accompanied by a 52 percent increase in circulating pesticides. By the twelve-month follow-up test, the participants who'd had surgery had lost 46 percent of their presurgery weight, but their pesticide levels had shot up 388 percent. Other studies confirm the phenomenon: weight loss and sky-rocketing pesticide levels go hand in hand.

These studies show very clearly that just releasing toxins from the fat into the bloodstream isn't enough to get them to leave your body. Instead, the toxins can actually flood your veins in higher levels, waiting for your body to reduce its lipolysis rate so they can go back into storage. Animal products with a high fat content are the most common sources of fat-soluble toxins, so if you're eating a diet high in animal fat, you're probably eating a lot of persistent organic pollutants.

As Jackie and many of my other patients have learned the hard way, this greater toxic presence doesn't just make and keep you fat. It can take a toll on many of your body's systems and tissues, not to mention the damage it does to your mitochondria. In an animal study that re-created the yo-yo diet effect, researchers found that when the animals were losing weight, the levels of the potent neurotoxin and immunotoxin hexachlorobenzene (HCB) rose dramatically in their blood and their brains—weight loss increased the concentration of HCB in fat tissue. The study also found that repeated weight loss and gain resulted in higher levels of HCB and fat in the liver. And, in turn, this fatty liver condition is associated with other health problems, including diabetes. HCB is also associated with symptoms such as headache, brain fog, and depression in humans. If you've already given up on diets, give yourself a big pat on the back for figuring out that *diet* is a four-letter word for a good reason.

Researchers have found that dieting without detoxing is one of the best ways to poison yourself and get fatter. In a study at Laval University, in Quebec, scientists showed that the rise in circulating toxins during weight loss led to a drop in the resting metabolic rate, which controls the number of calories burned when the body is at rest. The drop was caused by a reduction in the circulating level of the most active thyroid hormone, T_3. When T_3 levels are low, the likely results are low body temperature, fatigue, and weight gain. And after the diet is over, it is hard to keep the weight from coming back. As someone who had been dieting since she was a child, Jackie knew all too well that the fatigue is also likely to linger, and it may be accompanied by depression. The key is to take off the weight the right way, once and for all. That's the only way to live lean and head off or reverse obesity-related illnesses such as diabetes.

Conquering Diabetes

Eliminating toxins can also reverse one of the most troubling conditions that's on the rise: diabetes. Many scientific studies show a strong correlation between toxic burden and risk of type 2 diabetes. And since diabetes and being overweight go hand in hand, I'm convinced that a higher toxic burden and a higher body weight are also connected.

Being overweight is a main risk factor for diabetes, and diabetes is also associated with having persistent organic pollutants in your body. For people with high blood levels of fat-soluble toxins, the risk factor for developing diabetes goes up by an odds ratio of between 14 and 38. An odds ratio of 1 means you have the same risk ratio as everyone else to become diabetic; a ratio of 2 means you're twice as likely to become diabetic; so a ratio between 14 and 38 is astronomically high.

In addition, if soft drinks, cookies, and other sugar-filled products are part of your daily bread, you're increasing your odds of developing adult-onset diabetes that much more. The disease has been strongly associated with the consumption of sugar, and while FDA testing has consistently shown that refined sugar is free of toxins (and everything else except sucrose), the results are the same as if it were loaded with toxins. Chronic high sugar intake outpaces both insulin production and the cells' ability to respond to the insulin that's present.

Insulin is the means by which sugar is able to enter a cell from the bloodstream in order to nourish the cell. Most people with adult-onset diabetes actually have adequate insulin production, but their cells have become insensitive to the insulin. When that happens, they can have plenty of sugar in the bloodstream but the cells (including the brain cells) are starved of sugar. Not only does the sugar fail to make it into the cells where it's needed, but the extra sugar in the bloodstream can damage tissue. And much like toxins, sugar works against the liver's efforts to clear chemicals out of the bloodstream and prepare them for excretion. So having a low-sugar diet can go a long way toward preventing the problems that lead to diabetes.

Another culprit behind diabetes and many other chronic diseases is the mitochondrial dysfunction discussed earlier in this chapter. While there's ongoing debate among scientists as to which comes first—the dysfunction or the diabetes—there's no doubt that the two are connected.

What it all adds up to is that when you eat foods that are high in sugar and fat—the standard American diet—or one that's simply deficient in nutrients, you'll retain more toxins. When you eat a high-protein, low-fat, low-carb diet, you'll clear chemicals from your bloodstream more rapidly. But to avoid your toxic enemies, you need to know what they are and how they get into your home and your body. In chapter 2, you'll learn about the worst of these obesity-promoting villains, and you'll also find out that the worst effects of toxins are avoidable. While you can't elude them altogether, you can limit your exposure.

CHAPTER 2

The Toxin–Fat Connection

By the time my new patient Jeff found his way to my office, he was 70 pounds overweight and had multiple aches and pains and absolutely no energy, and he said he couldn't think as clearly or quickly as he used to. Routine medical tests had failed to find the cause of his problems, and he felt like a guinea pig with doctors putting him through a battery of tests and drugs. Although his excess weight had been his biggest complaint for years, now that his body was seemingly out of control, being overweight was the least of his concerns. Jeff was sure he was dying—and he was only forty years old.

In addition to being obese, Jeff was suffering from fatigue, depression, chronic infections, and headaches. He also had poor memory and felt shaky and off balance.

He said he'd started putting on the extra pounds in his twenties when he got his first desk job. Since then, he'd tried everything to lose weight, but nothing worked. Most of the people he knew had put on a few pounds over the years, so he thought it was just a normal part of getting older. Granted, he knew his case was more extreme, but after trying many different diets, he'd resigned himself to being heavy and was mostly trying to hold the line. He wasn't surprised when I said I was looking forward to seeing him drop some of that excess baggage, but he was surprised when I didn't put him on a diet as his previous doctors had done. I explained to Jeff that I suspected that his obesity and other problems stemmed from something else.

To figure out what it was, the first thing I did was spend a little time getting to know him. It was obvious from what he wrote on his chart and what he'd said so far that doctors had tried to treat his individual symptoms without trying to find out why he had all of these different symptoms and what it all meant. One of the keys to an accurate diagnosis is to keep looking for causes underlying symptoms until a pattern begins to emerge. Without a holistic view and understanding of the mind and body, this approach just isn't possible. Treating the symptoms without addressing the cause is like pulling the heads off dandelions instead of digging up the deep taproots. In no time, the dandelions will flower again because the roots are still in the ground. For Jeff to have energy, lose weight, and think clearly again, we had to get to the root of his problems. If I gave my patients natural remedies to take care of their symptoms and didn't identify and treat the cause, they'd never get better. They'd have to keep coming back for more remedies while their overall health continued to deteriorate. This would be a good thing for me if my goal were to get them into my office as often as possible, but I'd much rather help them get healthy and fit and stay that way. And the only way to do that is to deal with the cause of the excess weight or illness or both.

As a naturopathic physician, I need to be a sleuth. People are more than sets of symptoms, and I need to compile a complete picture of each patient as the whole person that he or she is. Once I get that big picture, I can order the right diagnostic tests and suggest a natural treatment. This takes time and focus; it doesn't happen with a fifteen-minute visit. So many patients tell me that their previous doctors assumed that their chronic fatigue, brain fog, and other symptoms were caused by lack of exercise, eating too much, or eating the wrong things. That assumption keeps doctors from looking deeply enough to discover the truth: that their patients are being poisoned.

As for Jeff's case, his chief complaints painted the classic picture of toxic overload. But I needed much more information. I needed to assess all of his symptoms and learn more about where he lived and worked, what he ate, and generally how he lived his life. This is the only way I could pinpoint which toxins were plaguing him, and then treat him accordingly.

I decided to run a blood test that detects the presence of the most common chlorinated pesticides. These pesticides kill bugs by knocking out the nervous system. In humans, the pesticides cause brain problems and can disable the immune system and upset hormonal balance—throwing two strikes at any attempt to lose weight. Autopsies have shown high levels of chlorinated pesticides in the fat of people with diseases such as heart disease, cirrhosis, metastatic liver disease, cerebral hemorrhage, hypertension, and cancer.

When the results of Jeff's tests came back, my suspicions were confirmed: Jeff had nine of the eighteen pesticides measured in this test.

Pesticides Hurt More Than the Pest

The load of pesticides circulating in Jeff's body was shocking enough in itself, but when you consider that the Environmental Protection Agency (EPA) has registered about 80,000 chemicals for daily use in this country and we have tests to check for only about 250 of them, it's truly unsettling to imagine what else Jeff—or any of us—might have. And the list of chemicals we're exposed to doesn't end at 80,000. Thousands of even more toxic chemicals are being used in countries that have less stringent regulations than ours. These chemicals eventually drift back to us in our air, our water, and our food. Ignorance may be bliss, but when it comes to toxins, it can be fattening and, in some cases, fatal.

One of the toxins in Jeff's blood was DDT, the chemical pesticide banned in 1977 thanks to the publication of *Silent Spring*, Rachel Carson's brilliant 1962 exposé of the effects of DDT and other persistent pesticides. How could Jeff have such a high level of a substance we haven't legally used in this country since he was eleven years old? DDT breaks down within six months of entering the body and turns into a different version of the beast, called DDE. Jeff had that, too, so it wasn't a one-time DDT exposure we were dealing with. But how could this be? He hadn't taken any trips out of the country. As it turned out, he didn't need to. Instead of going to the DDT, the DDT had come to him.

While DDT is banned for use in this country, it's still manufactured here and shipped to other countries for use in agriculture and mosquito control. In addition, most of the U.S. chemical companies have built plants in these other countries, where they make the pesticides for local use. No shipping required. Nice, huh? DDT then makes its way back to us in the agricultural products grown and raised in these countries and via the winds that blow around the planet.

A very disturbing statistic is that less than 1 percent of the pesticides that are sprayed actually make it to the target pest. That means more than 99 percent of all of the billions of pounds of pesticides that are sprayed don't affect the insect that's eating the crop. It's hard to imagine a more inefficient system. Would any sports team keep an athlete who made only 1 percent of his plays? If you've been waging a losing battle with your weight, you can be sure that some of those pesticides are in your body.

Despite the information that *Silent Spring* brought to light, the number of pesticides in use in the United States has risen from two hundred to eighteen thousand since its publication. We've gone from using 400 million pounds of the stuff in a year to using 4.5 billion pounds a year. The amount of pesticides used on our agricultural crops continues to double every ten years, and people continue to get fatter on pesticide-laden food that they think is healthy. Adding to this insanity, the insects become immune to many of these chemicals over time, and the number of insect species that cause crop damage actually increases! Plus, when we upset the natural order and kill off the main insect pests, other insects take over their turf. From 1970 to the early eighties, the number of species that cause crop damage — officially called pests — rose from ten to more than three hundred.

If this trend continues — and it will as long as we continue to support these toxic operations by buying nonorganic foods — one shudders to think what the produce will look and taste like, and what it will cost.

Over the past five decades the industrial chemical business has grown from a $2 billion industry to a $635 billion industry, and it continues to expand. According to the most recent EPA report,

4.4 billion pounds of industrial chemicals are released into the environment during the manufacturing process every year. Now, just where are those compounds ending up? They aren't disappearing—this isn't a magic show. And they don't evaporate. If you want to know where the toxins are ending up, look in the mirror. These chemicals are hiding out with your excess pounds of fat. And by the way, people who are slim can have just as many toxic chemicals hiding out in their bodies—their fat just has higher concentrations of them.

They've Got Us Surrounded

Along with pesticides, Jeff—like all of us—had encountered toxins from car exhaust, industrial solvents, plasticizers, paint, and household cleaning products on a daily basis. Every time he ate, drank, or took a breath, he was taking in a tiny amount of pollutants and poisons. A little new car smell here, a little spring fresh laundry detergent there, some rush hour exhaust fumes, a tuna melt microwaved in plastic wrap, a side of pesticide-glazed strawberries. Jeff's body had become a cesspool of polysyllabic substances, substances nature had never intended to be there.

Even if we could eliminate toxins from our environment entirely, there's still the fact that—are you ready for this?—we're *born* with a toxic burden. Toxins can be passed from mother to child. In 2004, the nonprofit Environmental Working Group (EWG) examined the cord blood, which circulates between a baby and its mother's placenta, of ten infants born in U.S. hospitals to study how many toxins are passed on. The results were startling: EWG researchers found that newborns begin their lives with exposure to as many as 287 of the 413 toxic chemicals being studied. An average of 200 toxins were found per baby, and 101 toxins were found in all of the babies. The 287 toxins included 180 chemical compounds that have been shown to cause cancer in either animals or humans. (Incidentally, all chemicals that cause cancer in humans were initially found to cause it in animals.) The babies also had 217 compounds that damage the central nervous system, and 208 compounds that lead to developmental problems. And who knows what happens when these chemicals work together? No one has studied the effects of those toxic combinations yet.

As parents, we all hope to pass on to our children our most wonderful traits. Most of us don't think about or count on passing on a load of toxins. When mothers find out about it, most of them feel guilty ("What have I done to my child?"). Yet it's a sad fact of living in a toxic world, and it happens with all mammals on the planet. If I were able to influence the young women of the world, I'd ask them all to get tested to measure their toxic burden and then go through the cleansing program before they conceive. While you may not have a say in the eye color of your child, you can change the toxic load you're passing on.

Because compounds such as DDT weren't used agriculturally or residentially until the 1940s, mothers of baby boomers accumulated only a few years' worth of them. Their daughters started with that small amount and added to it every day with their exposure to contaminated air, food, and water. By the time the daughters became pregnant, they'd amassed a greater total burden than their mothers had and passed some of it to the next generation. Those children then started life with an even greater toxin load than their parents had and much more than their grandparents had. A few years ago, I treated a family who had three generations of lead toxicity, with the toxin passing from mother to daughter to grandson.

Toxic Connections

- Obesity rates have more than doubled in the past thirty years among children aged two to five and twelve to nineteen, and they've more than tripled among those aged six to eleven.
- The asthma rate among children rose from 3.6 percent to 8.7 percent from 1980 to 2001.
- The preterm birth rate increased 23 percent in the twenty years from 1984 to 2004 (the United States has the highest rate in the world).
- The childhood cancer rate has risen 67.1 percent since 1950 (the United States has the fourth-highest rate in the world).

And once we're born, without doing anything unusual, we go on to accumulate tiny traces of poison every day. Persistent organic pollutants are in the air we breathe, indoors and out, and in the food we eat and the beverages we drink, including water. They're in our soil—our backyards and our gardens. They're in the refrigerator and in the pantry. They're in the garage, under the kitchen sink, on laundry room shelves, in the dust particles in our ventilation ducts, and around our TVs and stereos. And they're in our medicine cabinets—in soaps, lotions, and makeup. They all have names like "2-(diethylamino)-6-methylpyridin-4-yl/one," so you know they mean business.

People chalk up a lot of their symptoms to getting older, but it's not because we're adding years—it's because we're adding significant amounts of toxins every year. Studies have found that the levels of pesticides in people's blood prior to dieting and stomach stapling correlate with age, not weight: the most pesticides are in the oldest people, not the heaviest. Since toxins bioaccumulate over time, lingering and gathering in fat cells, this finding makes perfect sense.

One of the most extensive studies of Americans' toxic burden was funded by the EWG and conducted at the Mount Sinai School of Medicine. In 1992, the EWG tested nine adults, none of whom worked in industries that would expose them to high levels of environmental poisons. One was an international organic-farming activist, and another was the well-known journalist Bill Moyers. All nine were tested for the presence of 210 contaminants internationally recognized to be persistent pollutants—many of them fat-soluble compounds such as DDT. The results: their blood and urine showed the presence of 167 of the 210 contaminants, with an average of 91 in any given person.

Each person tested had an average of

- 53 chemicals that have been linked to cancer;
- 62 compounds toxic to the central nervous system (including the brain);
- 58 compounds toxic to the endocrine (hormonal) system;
- 55 compounds that are toxic to the immune system and typically lead to autoimmunity and impaired ability to fight infections.

True multitaskers, these chemicals. The study led Moyers to do a documentary on the chemical industry, but *Trade Secrets* received very little publicity and, to my knowledge, was never aired again. But if you can find a copy, I highly recommend you watch it. You can also find a transcript of it at www.pbs.org/tradesecrets/transcript.html.

In the past several years, most of my new patients have shown up with toxin-caused ailments such as allergies, asthma, diabetes, chemical sensitivities, fibromyalgia, infertility, Parkinsonism, bone

---

Nine Classes of Toxic Compounds That Weigh Everyone Down, No Exceptions

1. Dioxins—four different dioxins (commonly thought of as the most toxic of all synthetic compounds) have been found in all people studied. These toxins are contaminants produced when chlorine-containing compounds are made in chemical plants.
2. Volatile and semivolatile compounds—solvents including:
   * Styrene
   * Xylene
   * Dichlorobenzene
   * Ethylphenol
3. Halogenated compounds, including those that contain either chlorine or bromine, such as:
   * DDE/T, PCBs, chlordanes—chlorinated pesticides
   * PBDE (flame retardants)
4. Organophosphate pesticides.
5. Phthalates in plastics.
6. Naphthalenes.
7. Polycyclic aromatic hydrocarbons from combustion sources.
8. Heavy metals, including:
   * Lead—Pb
   * Mercury—Hg
   * Cadmium—Cd
   * Arsenic—As
9. Bisphenol A.

marrow cancers—lymphomas, leukemias, and multiple myeloma—and autoimmune diseases such as lupus, rheumatoid arthritis, and Hashimoto's thyroiditis. Sadly, this laundry list of toxin-caused sickness is growing like a weed. Millions of people who don't know that toxins can make them fat and sick have no idea why they can't lose weight or why they feel so lousy. Those who are aware of this connection worry that it's only a matter of time before they ingest or inhale the chemical straw that breaks the camel's back. Many of my patients want to point to one specific toxin and say, "This is what made me sick." In most cases, that exposure was merely the one that tipped the toxic scales. The most recent exposure adds to the total burden they've been accumulating all of their lives and pushes the load over the top.

Although this picture may look bleak, if you're armed with the right information, you absolutely can live a lean and healthy life. A growing number of us know that living clean and green is the smart thing to do, but for many this concept just sounds like a passing trend being promoted by health nuts or environmentalists. Most people are so used to eating, drinking, and breathing toxins that it feels normal and natural to them. The irony here is that being clean and green is what nature intended and the only way for us to be physically fit and mentally balanced.

As Jackie and Jeff discovered firsthand, obesity and many other conditions and illnesses can be completely reversed by countering the effects of toxins. I'm happy to say I've seen all of the above illnesses and symptoms improve in my patients as they followed the four-week plan in chapter 7. You may be most excited about fitting back into your favorite jeans or losing your double chin, but when you start to wake up with energy and feel good again, you'll realize that as great as looking good is, feeling great is even better.

Waiter, There's a Toxin in My Soup

You can't always have control over the invisible toxins in your midst, but you can control the amount of toxins you put in your mouth. So one of the first things I ask patients like Jeff to do is to learn which foods have the greatest toxin burdens and which have the smallest. As a traveling salesman in the Pacific Northwest, he ate out most of the time and was limited to what was on the menu wherever he happened to stop.

> ### Leading Sources of Chlorinated Pesticides
> - Nonorganic beef
> - Nonorganic dairy products
> - Farm-raised fish (especially salmon and catfish)
> - Nonorganic butter

We're on Our Own

Right about now you might be wondering how this all got started in the first place and why it's been allowed to go on. Why haven't all of these chemicals been tested for harmful effects? The fact is that chemicals have made our lives easier in many ways, and we all know how great the demand for convenience is in America. Overburdened government agencies can't do all of the testing themselves. They can do very little of it, in fact, so they're left to take the word of manufacturers—manufacturers with the money to sway public opinion by hiring product-defense experts, PR firms, and lawyers.

Most people think the government wouldn't allow companies to expose consumers to toxins in air, food, or water. After all, we have the EPA and the Food and Drug Administration. Aren't they supposed to watch out for us? The sad truth is we can't rely on government and captains of industry to protect us. They aren't championing our health. Even when government agencies do attempt to head off the use of harmful substances, they face expensive, time-consuming battles. What's worse, some of the agencies are run by people who have come out of the very industries they're supposed to be regulating.

Because cause and effect is so difficult to establish when it comes to the harm that chemicals can do, scientists tend to stay out of it. The current scientific method calls for researchers to try to identify the impact of a single agent on health. But our health problems come from a total burden of hundreds of toxic compounds, and our accepted scientific method doesn't even begin to address this type of problem. It's just not as simple as finding that everyone with a certain illness has had one specific virus or bacteria. In addition, funding is limited. So for the time being, research money seems destined to go mostly to curing illness rather than to preventing it by focusing on the toxins causing so much of it. That makes it our responsibility to be aware of the dangers out there.

Once Jeff was armed with the information I'd given him, he began to be more careful about what he ordered at restaurants and what he bought at the grocery store. He also started taking supplements to help rid himself of fat-soluble toxins more efficiently than he could manage on his own. (I'll cover the best supplements for this purpose in chapter 6 and tell you exactly which supplements to take and how much in week four of the four-week plan.) Jeff was so toxic that he needed to use all of his body's detox organs and exit routes, so he also took regular saunas to sweat toxins out and underwent colonic irrigations.

I have to hand it to Jeff for doing the work to regain his health. So many patients come in wanting me to just give them a pill to make them better so that they can get back to living their lives the way they had been. Making the effort to change the way they eat and generally cleanse their bodies (on the inside) is rarely at the top of their to-do lists. But Jeff listened to what I had to say and then followed my advice even though if he'd sought a second opinion, he almost certainly wouldn't have found another doctor who would have agreed with me at that time.

Like so many of my patients, Jeff just needed more information. He thought he was being relatively healthy, because he didn't have accurate information and he hadn't been given any good options. When he understood what was happening with his body and realized that it was up to him to take his health back, he made an "I love my body" lifestyle change.

It didn't take long to notice improvements in his health. Once he grew accustomed to the new routine, he lost 20 pounds in just two months with absolutely no changes to his overall diet. He avoided foods known to have high toxic burdens, but he didn't have to make any sacrifices—he just bought clean organic versions of the same foods he'd been eating. This is something that astonishes most of my patients. It seems too easy to be true, but it's evidence of how damaging toxins are and how healthy clean green food is for every cell in your body.

As the toxins cleared from Jeff's body, his mitochondria were able to start doing their job again. Within weeks, the looming fear that he was dying faded from his mind. He quickly regained his energy and his brain function, and, best of all, he started to enjoy life and have fun again.

If he can do it, so can you. It starts with awareness of what's inside your body and how it's getting there.

An Apple a Day Won't Keep the Doctor Away—Unless It's Organic

Part of my job as a naturopathic physician specializing in environmental medicine is to teach my patients where the dangers lurk and how to be healthy and live lean in a toxic, fattening world. Who would have predicted that the "apple a day" adage would be reversed by something called organophosphate pesticides?

These pesticides are used on vegetables and fruit, and unless you wash the heck out of nonorganic produce, you're having pesticides for dinner. Some pesticides have been banned, but others are still in use for both indoor and outdoor pest control. And they're hard to avoid. Notice how you never see bugs in grocery stores, hotels, restaurants, or movie theaters? They're sprayed every day. Studies have shown that children who live in homes where organophosphate pesticides—the most commonly used class of pesticides—are used have a higher rate of brain tumors. People usually have no idea that the compounds they're sprinkling on their roses to kill aphids or spraying under the sink for ants can have such serious consequences.

Pesticides were one of the things working against Jackie while she was proudly getting her recommended "five a day" of fruits and vegetables. She was a smart and motivated woman who ate a diet high in fruits and vegetables and low in red meats—just what I typically recommend—but when I asked her whether her produce was organic, the plot thickened. Like so many people, she had the notion that organic foods were just another way to get people to spend more money and really weren't so different from regular food.

It is true that some nonorganic veggies and fruits are less toxic than others, but the ones that are high in toxins were among Jackie's favorites. She was also buying meats and dairy products that contained chlorinated pesticides, which have been documented to slow thermo-genesis—the rate at which our fats are burned to make energy—making it hard to lose weight and easy to gain it. The higher the pesticide levels in your blood, the slower you burn calories while you're sleeping (when most of a given day's calories are burned) and while you're sedentary. If you have a low rate of thermogenesis, you tend to have more body fat. When your metabolism returns to normal, you'll burn more calories while you're resting and sleeping, and you'll have less fat.

The effect chlorinated pesticides have on thermogenesis was also revealed in a study that gauged how efficiently mitochondria use fatty acids for fuel. The higher the blood levels of pesticides and PCBs were, the less fatty acids were burned. This means that besides burning fewer calories, a person will be more likely to gain weight and have a very hard time losing it.

Another reason that nonorganic apples aren't so healthy anymore is that they're typically grown in soil that's been degraded by these pesticides and toxic fertilizers. Soil that's been degraded produces crops that are nutritionally lacking. This isn't my opinion—it's a fact. The U.S. Department of Agriculture (USDA) has reported that the nutrient content of American produce has declined significantly since the 1950s, when use of these chemicals became commonplace. Organic foods often have more minerals and phytochemicals than conventionally grown produce—a result of having to work harder to fend off disease and pests. In doing so, they produce more healthy compounds than their conventional, nonorganic, counterparts produce.

And the shortcomings of conventional produce may have a connection to obesity and chronic diseases, including cancer. Bruce Ames, a biochemist and molecular biologist at the University of California, Berkeley, found that insufficiencies of vitamins and minerals can damage DNA, which opens the door to cancer. He also believes that these deficiencies can prompt people to overeat as their bodies desperately try to gain the nutrients they're not getting.

What is your health worth? What is it worth to feel vital every day? What is it worth to have a body that you're proud of and that works the way you want it to? Buying nonorganic food may have saved Jackie some money in the checkout lane, but then again it may not have. When you add up how much money she'd spent on physicians before seeing me or how much she'd spent to get the pesticides out of her body, nonorganic food becomes the more expensive choice.

Jackie, who had been so proud of her five servings a day of fruits and vegetables, was furious when she found that not only was she paying for pesticides that were making her fat, but she was also getting only a small fraction of the nutrients she thought she was getting. For her, that was incentive enough to go organic, regardless of the cost.

The EWG recently studied extensive USDA and FDA testing that measured pesticide residues in produce and then ranked the most commonly eaten fruits and vegetables in this country on a scale from most toxic to most consistently clean. I strongly encourage you to take the list of the "dirty dozen" to the grocery store with you. If your produce manager isn't stocking organic versions of all of the following, you may want to enlighten him or her.

The Dirty Dozen (highest in pesticides)
Apples
Bell peppers
Carrots
Celery
Cherries
Grapes (imported)
Kale
Lettuce
Nectarines
Peaches
Pears
Strawberries

What a conundrum. We know we're supposed to eat our fruit and vegetables because they have crucial nutrients that other foods don't, but here on the dirty dozen list, some of our favorites are covered with the most toxic agricultural chemicals out there. So do yourself and your family a favor and buy these twelve only if they're organically grown. And eat a good variety, because they all contain different antioxidants.

If you can't find organic and you're determined to eat the forbidden fruit (or vegetable), the nonorganic varieties can sometimes be

Detoxing Nonorganic Produce

If you can't find organic varieties, use these methods to reduce your toxic exposure:

- Use a vegetable peeler to remove the skin from commercial varieties of apples, pears, nectarines, and potatoes. You'll probably need a paring knife to peel peaches.
- For bell peppers, apples, and celery, use an acid wash:
  1. Fill a large bowl or a plastic food storage container with water.
  2. Add a cup of distilled vinegar.
  3. Let the produce rest in the tub for ten to twenty-five minutes, and then use a vegetable scrub brush to scrub each piece for about sixty seconds.
  4. For grapes and cherries, just let them soak for about sixty minutes.

made less toxic by peeling them (great for apples and potatoes, not so great for lettuce and strawberries). Their toxic content can be further reduced by soaking and scrubbing them in a tub of 10 percent vinegar (also not so great for lettuce and strawberries). And regardless of whether it's organic or nonorganic, wash it. Whatever it is that's keeping the bugs at bay at the supermarket is also surely settling on the surface of the produce.

Avoiding the nonorganic versions altogether is the best strategy, though. A study in Seattle showed that when the most toxic fruits and vegetables were removed from preschoolers' diets (along with almonds) and replaced with organic varieties, the kids' pesticide levels went way down. Their levels of key pesticides dropped to essentially zero and stayed undetectable until they started eating conventional foods again.

So now that you know what not to eat, what should you eat? You can start with the flip side of the dirty dozen: the clean dozen. Not all nonorganic versions of fruits and vegetables pack a toxic punch, and these twelve have virtually no pesticide levels. These are the nonor-ganic varieties you can buy without lying awake at night regretting that you've made your toxic burden worse.

The Clean Dozen (lowest in pesticides)
Asparagus
Avocados
Cabbage
Eggplant
Kiwis
Mangoes
Onions
Papayas
Pineapples
Sweet corn
Sweet peas
Watermelon

While it would obviously be best to buy organic varieties of all of our foods, when it comes to these twelve fruits and vegetables, you can feel safe buying the commercial varieties. So unless you have a big grocery budget that allows you to buy nothing but organic foods, use your organic allowance to buy organic apples instead of organic broccoli or bananas.

PCBs Span the Globe

Another major source of our toxic burden is PCBs—polychlorinated biphenyls—a highly toxic chemical cocktail found in all of the adults and in the cord blood of all of the newborns who have been studied in the United States. In fact, PCBs have been found in the fat of everyone tested around the globe. Originally manufactured for use as coolants in electrical transformers, PCBs went on to serve many other industrial uses. They've thoroughly contaminated our environment, and they've contaminated us as well with effects both visible and invis-ible. They cause mitochondrial dysfunction, which as you've learned contributes to weight gain, and the very visible result is fat. But the invisible damage they can do to the immune system and the brain is far more insidious and sometimes cancer causing. Because PCBs are found in people, animals, fish, and soil throughout the world—and because of their clearly documented health effects—a worldwide ban on PCB production has been in effect since the 1970s. But that doesn't mean we can breathe easy. We're born with PCBs in our system, and rather than break down, they simply persist in our bodies. It's the same story with all of the animals of the world, and as well as passing on the burden through reproduction, they pass it on when they're eaten. Yes, the circle of life gets more toxic as the world turns.

Studies conducted among the Arctic Inuit have linked their traditional diet of local fish and game to elevated blood levels of PCBs and increased rates of ear infection. In fact, some samples of Inuit breast milk have far exceeded the levels of these compounds that would be allowed in commercial cow's milk or baby formula.

The concentration of PCBs in the Arctic may be higher than in most other places because of a phenomenon called leapfrogging. The process begins at the equator, where the higher temperatures turn PCBs into vapor. In that form, the PCBs ride the wind both northward and southward. At night when the temperature drops, these chemicals become liquid again and land on the soil, plants, and water. When the sun comes up the next morning and heats the earth, the PCBs can revolatize and rise back into the air to travel on the wind again toward the north and south poles. When they near the poles, where the environment is cool, they're less able to revolatize. As a result, the soil, plants, and animals nearest the poles become more toxic with these compounds. And as with the Inuit, PCBs bioaccumulate in the people who eat these plants and animals.

When trying to assess levels of PCB exposure in certain areas, butter is a good place to look. It is fat-soluble and allows chemists to monitor how PCBs are being spread around the planet, starting with cattle feed making its way into the cow, then into the milk and the meat, and ultimately into human stomachs. But PCBs also spread through air and water, and the study of butter has revealed a bioaccumulation in cows. In global samplings of butter, the highest levels of PCBs have been found in butter made in Europe and North America.

In North America, fish is the other top source of PCBs, with farmed Atlantic salmon being the single greatest source. Though wild salmon's health benefits are well known, farmed salmon is a vastly different story.

A study by the Food Safety Authority of Ireland found that farmed salmon has an average of four times more PCBs, dioxins, and other persistent chlorinated contaminants than wild salmon. Though this study was done on a relatively small number of fish, it was backed up by later studies. In one study, researchers tested more than seven hundred salmon totaling about 2 metric tons of farmed and wild salmon from around the globe. The results: Thirteen persistent chlorinated pollutants were found in significantly higher levels in farmed salmon than in wild salmon.

Farmed salmon has significantly higher levels of PCBs, dioxins, and the chlorinated pesticides toxaphene and dieldrin than wild Alaskan salmon. Even the least contaminated farmed-fish samples, from Washington State and Chile, have much higher levels of PCBs, dioxins, and dieldrin than their wild counterparts. The most contaminated farmed salmon comes from Scotland and the Faeroe Islands, in the North Atlantic.

Researchers also tested the fish pellets that these farmed salmon were fed and found the source of the contamination: other fish. The feed pellets are made from small fish that have been contaminated with PCBs, which then build up in the salmon to levels that are twenty to thirty times higher than what's found in their natural food sources in the wild. Unfortunately, cooking doesn't reduce the levels, and the PCBs are transferred directly into the bodies of consumers.

The risks posed by this level of PCB contamination are especially serious for the children of women who ate these fish while pregnant. Studies in Michigan, North Carolina, and Taiwan have shown that children exposed to PCBs while in utero have more cognitive defects, poorer gross motor function, and less visual memory than those who weren't exposed. These studies are ongoing, and the neurological effects, including lower IQ levels and behavioral problems like ADHD, are still being found in the children during their teen years.

Clearly, eating farmed salmon poses serious risks. Neurotoxic effects have even been documented in adults who ate Great Lakes fish with high PCB levels. Among Lake Michigan fish eaters, those with the highest blood levels of PCBs also had the most problems with learning and memory.

When I shared this information with Jeff, he was incredulous. For years he'd been going out of his way to eat salmon once a week. He had no idea that the farmed version he'd been buying was contributing to his illness, not to his health.

Don't Eat the Big Fish

As upset as Jeff was to learn that farmed salmon was doing him more harm than good, he was equally disturbed to learn that his other favorite fish—tuna and swordfish—were adding mercury to his toxic burden.

Because mercury is very slow to leave the body, regular consumption of high-mercury fish makes for long-term exposure. It takes close to 70 days for the dose of mercury from a tuna sandwich to drop by 50 percent in an adult's bloodstream (mercury is present in all tuna—canned, fresh, whatever). It takes another 70 days for it to drop to 25 percent, another 70 days for it to reach 12.5 percent (we're now at 210 days after the sandwich) and another 70 days for the blood level to reach 6.75 percent of the original dose. It takes a whole year to get the blood levels down to zero, but even then you're not out of the woods—mercury's half-life (the time it takes for a chemical to be reduced by half) in the brain is about 20 years. At that kind of price, you'd better have enjoyed that sandwich.

Like PCBs, mercury has been found in all of the newborns and adults tested. This heavy metal and most of its compounds are extremely toxic. The major sources of exposure are high-mercury fish and silver dental amalgams used for fillings, which are half mercury by weight.

If someone is eating any of the high-mercury fish regularly, his or her blood level of this powerful neurotoxin (and immunotoxin) can be quite high. Blood levels of mercury are often found to be elevated in consumers of high-end fish such as swordfish and halibut.

This is shocking when you consider that "normal" blood levels of mercury and other heavy metals are based on industrial-exposure standards. When we exceed these standards, our mercury levels are in the range associated with adverse health effects. If Jeff had been exposed to the level of mercury we found in his body while on a job in an industrial setting, he'd have been sent home and not allowed to return to work until his levels had dropped. That's how much mercury he had accumulated.

Mercury enters the environment as a pollutant by way of various industries, especially coal-fired power suppliers. It's also introduced through the disposal of certain products such as auto parts, fluorescent lightbulbs, and medical products. Fish pick up mercury when water carrying this substance passes over their gills. Fish don't have an efficient means of clearing mercury from their bodies, so it builds up to a very high level. In addition to what they get from the water, big fish eating smaller fish absorb the entire load of mercury that the smaller fish had eaten during its lifetime. In other words, the big fish adds the small fish's mercury buildup to its own. (The half-life for methylmercury in fish is two years.) Since saltwater fish such as tuna and swordfish can live longer and grow to very large sizes, their levels of mercury can reach exceptionally high levels. Although Jackie had initially told me she felt guilty for not eating much fish, she was happy to hear that by avoiding the big fish, she'd done herself a favor.

You'll probably be surprised to learn that in addition to certain fish and dental fillings, mercury compounds can be found in over-the-counter drugs, including topical antiseptics, stimulant laxatives, diaper-rash ointment, eyedrops, and nasal sprays. The FDA maintains that it has "inadequate data to establish general recognition of the safety and effectiveness" of the mercury ingredients in these products. So buyer beware.

How Fattening Can a Container Be?

What do most Americans eat many times every day? The first time I heard this question I guessed candy. The correct answer? Plastic.

The respected researcher Dr. Frederick von Saal recently oversaw a test for the *Milwaukee Journal Sentinel* in which he microwaved food in "microwave-safe" containers, including prepackaged frozen meals, soup, and baby food. He found that all of these containers transferred the estrogenic compound bisphenol A (BPA) to the foods. When the label on a plastic container says it's microwave safe, that doesn't mean it doesn't contaminate food with plastic during microwaving—it means the plastic container won't melt during the microwave session.

Microwaving foods in plastic increases the migration of plastic to the food the longer it's heated and the higher the temperature. While food in direct contact with the plastic sustains the greatest contamination during microwaving, the plastic molecules bounce all around and contaminate even the food that isn't in contact with the plastic. When I first met Jackie and Jeff, they were eating frozen microwaved dinners two or three times a week. Neither of them knew they were also eating plastic that contained hormones that could disrupt their bodies' natural balance.

Among plastics' drawbacks, they're known to be disrupters of the hormonal system and have been linked to premature sexual development in girls. Some types of plastic may also increase our risk of cancer. People who work in factories that manufacture plastic products have higher rates of certain cancers, including prostate cancers. And the substances added to plastics to make them soft or pliable pose another serious problem. Plasticizers can contaminate food through simple contact—they don't even need to be heated, though that certainly makes matters worse. Levels of plasticizers are high in store-wrapped meat, poultry, fish, and especially cheese, and the movement of plastics from plastic wrap to food increases with the length of time they're in contact with each other. The rate of "travel" is also greater if the food's fat content is high.

While eating plastic with your meals doesn't equal the level of plasticizers that plastic workers are exposed to, we don't know how much exposure is enough to cause cancers. So try to keep plastic out of your diet. While it's difficult to avoid buying food wrapped in plastic, you can leave plastic out of the food-heating process.

Some plastics also contain a common toxin associated with becoming diabetic. BPA is a component of polycarbonate plastic (recycling number 7), which is used in the ever-popular Nalgene drinking bottles, baby bottles, food containers, dental fillings, medical tubing, and the lining of metal food and beverage cans. A study of BPA's effect on human fat tissue revealed that it can cause the bodily changes that lead to obesity and resistance to insulin, both of which are major steps in the progression toward adult-onset diabetes. BPA has been shown to cause insulin resistance in mice and in all likelihood will one day be

Know the Numbers

The different kinds of plastics can be identified by the numbers stamped in the middle of the triangular recycling symbol.

Here are the less toxic ones:

1—polyethylene terephthalate (PET): used for single-use bottles and containers; recyclable

2—high-density polyethylene (HDPE): used for milk jugs, shampoo bottles, toys, etc.; recyclable

3—low-density polyethylene (LDPE): used for plastic wrap, grocery bags, etc.

4—polypropylene (PP): used for syrup and yogurt containers, diapers, etc.

Here are the more toxic ones:

5—polyvinyl chloride (PVC): used in cling wrap for packaged meats. Vinyl chloride is a known carcinogen. PVC also includes phthalates, which interfere with hormone development.

6—extruded polystyrene (PS): commonly known as Styrofoam. Styrene is considered a carcinogen.

7—polycarbonate (PC): used for baby bottles, watercooler jugs, and epoxy linings of tin cans. PC is composed of bisphenol A, which has been linked to cancer and obesity.

shown to cause the same problems in humans—at doses you're being exposed to right this very minute.

Breathing Can Make You Fat

If you feel like all you have to do is smell a doughnut to gain weight, you might actually be on to something. While the scent of the doughnut in itself can't make you fat, the other particles you inhale may do just that. All of the airborne toxins you're exposed to the most are associated with weight gain. Benzo(a)pyrene (BAP) from cigarettes, tailpipes, and other combustion sources has the ability to inhibit lipolysis in fat tissue. This fat breakdown is the necessary first step in the chain of events that ends with thermogenesis. The stored fat has to go through this process to be released into the bloodstream as free fatty acids. After release, they're transported into the cells and ushered to the mitochondria, where they're used as fuel. In addition to blocking the release of fatty acids from storage, BAP has been shown to actually cause weight gain in animals.

Obviously, anyone living in an urban or suburban area with lots of traffic will be exposed to BAP on a daily basis. Smokers, of course, will have even greater exposure. So it's more than just a sedentary lifestyle in the city that leads to obesity—it's also the air.

Chlorinated toxins' power to cause weight gain even spans generations. A recent study revealed that the levels of the chlorinated toxin HCB in a pregnant woman's body will influence her child's weight. The higher the mother's toxic level, the higher the risk that her child will be overweight or fall into the obese category. The children in this study were followed until they were six years old, so it's clear that their HCB exposure in the womb had long-term effects. In addition to being at risk for being overweight, these children have higher rates of behavior problems, including attention deficit (hyperactivity) disorder and poor social skills.

The EWG newborn study found that in addition to passing on chlorinated pesticides and PCBs to their children, mothers pass along toxins released by plastics, chemicals released by Teflon pans, and combustion byproducts from outdoor air pollution and smoking. In the study, unless the mother was a smoker or was exposed to secondhand smoke on a regular basis, most of the combustion byproducts came from outdoor air pollution created by cars and trucks (especially diesel vehicles), factories, and power plants. Teflon chemicals came from cooking with nonstick pans and eating food that was cooked in them.

And those air fresheners that people are liberally spraying throughout their homes are chock-full of solvents that are neurotoxins. Some air fresheners even have a drug-abuse warning on the side of the can because they're so high in solvents—they can be sprayed onto a rag and sniffed like glue. Once in the lungs, they immediately pass into the bloodstream and make their way throughout the body within seconds. When they reach the brain, they dampen its functioning the same way that having a few drinks would. And then there are the plug-in air fresheners that we see advertised on TV. Go to the store and look at the side of the box—another drug-abuse warning. Are we trying to make our families neurotoxic? If you have these in your house, throw them away. Otherwise, you're being poisoned one breath at a time.

And when it comes to solvent exposure, air fresheners aren't the only culprits. The greatest source is indoor smoking. Smoking also contributes combustion byproducts, cancer-causing chemicals, and heavy metals to the air. After cigarette smoke, the next-greatest sources of solvent exposure are carpeting, new cabinetry, and new paint. Cleaning supplies, including tile cleaners, have solvents, and so do dry-cleaned clothes. But Jackie was most surprised to find out that there are solvents in many perfumes, including her favorite.

Are you feeling surrounded? If you're getting the idea that airborne polluters are everywhere, you're right. Here's the lineup of major offenders:

- **Aromatic hydrocarbons.** These are byproducts of combustion that include benzo(a)pyrene (BAP) and naphthalenes. Sources include tailpipes, cigarettes, and smokestacks. In a 2000 study, 200 placentas were tested for the presence of the seven major aromatic hydrocarbons after the mothers had given birth. The researchers found that 199 of the 200 had all seven toxins (the other placenta had six). This means that our children are exposed to combustion chemicals that Mom breathes in during pregnancy. They disrupt the normal functioning of mitochondria, causing fatigue, obesity, and many other problems.
- **Arsenic.** This is a heavy-metal poison that's found naturally in groundwater and in high concentrations in cigarette smoke. Besides disrupting the mitochondria, it's known to cause cancer and diabetes. In 2001, the National Academy of Sciences reported that arsenic causes cancer in humans "at doses that are close to the drinking-water concentrations that occur in the United States."
- **Cadmium.** This is another common heavy metal that's found in high concentrations in cigarette smoke and is also in our food supply. It disrupts the mitochondria, causes cancer and kidney damage, and increases the risk of osteoporosis.

- **Dioxins.** These are poisonous petroleum-derived chemicals produced whenever chlorine is used industrially (in pesticide and herbicide production, for example, and in the bleaching of wood pulp for paper products) and when plastics are burned. These mitochondrial toxins are considered to be the most toxic synthetic chemicals known. They're known to cause birth defects, miscarriages, mutations, and the skin disease chloracne.
- **Furans.** These are flammable, volatile, and highly toxic liquids made from pine oils or manufactured synthetically and used in organic chemistry. These are also mitochondrial toxins but haven't been well studied in relation to adverse health effects.
- **Hexachlorobenzene (HCB).** This is a chlorinated hydrocarbon formerly used as a seed treatment, especially on wheat. After its introduction as a fungicide in 1945 for crop seeds, it was found in all food types and was banned from use in the United States in 1966. It is an animal carcinogen and is considered a probable human carcinogen. Chronic exposure in humans has been shown to adversely affect mitochondrial and neurological functions and lead to ailments including a liver disease (Porphyria cutanea tarda), skin lesions, ulcers, sensitivity to light, and hair loss. Human and animal studies have shown that HCB is one of the toxins that cross the placenta to accumulate in fetal tissues, and it's also transferred in breast milk. HCB is highly toxic to aquatic organisms.
- **Organophosphate pesticides.** These are the most commonly used class of pesticides, which kill insects by poisoning their nervous systems. These compounds came out of German research on nerve gases after World War I. Studies indicate that these potent mitochondrial toxins can kill brain cells and scramble synapses (nerve connections) in fetuses and children. They can also lead to childhood brain cancer.
- **Perfluorocarbons (PFCs).** These are powerful greenhouse gases used most commonly in refrigerators and in some cosmetics. They chip away at the ozone layer and appear to take a toll on our immune systems as well.

Now that you've been introduced to the toxic saboteurs that are stopping you from having the healthy body that you want, it's time to rid them from your life.

PART TWO

The Clean, Green Solution

CHAPTER 3

A Different Kind of Diet

Michelle, a forty-one-year-old accountant, came to me because she was desperate to lose weight. She said she had never lost the extra baggage after having her second baby and she'd been gaining 8 or 9 pounds every year since then, even though she watched what she ate. At 5 feet 6 inches and 235 pounds, she said she could barely keep up with her eleven- and thirteen-year-old daughters, and her husband was worried that if she didn't lose weight she might have a heart attack.

"I used to be embarrassed to be a size 14. Now I'd give anything to fit in that size again," she said. "What kind of a diet can you put me on that will really work?"

"How about a diet that isn't a diet?" I said. "Those are the only kind that really work."

I get a lot of interesting looks from patients when I say that, but Michelle looked at me with such suspicion that I had to smile. Patients who are willing to be totally honest with me about what they're thinking and feeling are the ones I can usually help the most.

I asked Michelle to tell me what else was going on with her health. She told me she was having allergic reactions that she hadn't had when she was younger. Until she was in her thirties, she was allergic only to ragweed and pollen. Her allergies had become worse over the years, and now everything from a dusty room to strong perfume could set off a coughing or sneezing attack. If she got stuck in an elevator with someone wearing clothes scented by a dryer sheet, she'd feel as if she were going to pass out. She said she also had digestive problems and felt tired all the time. "I don't even know why I bother to go to bed anymore. I swear I'm more tired when I get up the next day," she said.

Michelle's array of ailments, especially those with an autoimmune theme, signaled that her body had more of a toxic load than it could handle. If she could get rid of the toxins, she'd get rid of the fat they were stored in, too (not to mention all of the health problems that went along with them). The reason she had that fat in the first place was that she needed a place to store the toxins, and in a happy feedback loop, she'd let go of that weight as she let go of the toxins.

When I suggested that we start with lowering her body load of toxins, Michelle was puzzled at first. But as I explained the connection between toxins and her ailments, I could see excitement in her eyes. Realizing that all of her problems had a common cause, she felt the stirrings of hope for the first time in years.

My greatest lessons about being a physician all came after I'd graduated from naturopathic medical school. When I was in school, I learned about lots of health problems but never heard a word about multiple chemical sensitivities. I can't even recall anyone with this debilitating condition coming into the college clinic. But after starting a practice and making up my mind to believe whatever my patients told me about their health no matter how crazy it sounded, that's when my education really started. My stance might not sound especially revolutionary, but, relatively speaking, it is. In both standard and alternative medicine, there's a pervasive belief system that may be best summed up as, "If I haven't heard of it, it doesn't exist." Maybe you've run into this philosophy during visits with physicians, especially if you've been interested in naturopathic techniques and wanted to talk about them.

The first time a patient told me that whenever he was around a chemical odor he lost his brain function and felt exhausted for the rest of the day, I was utterly unable to understand the reason for this. But

I believed him (a great relief to him after getting nowhere with his regular doctor) and began to investigate how I could help him best. As I pursued this path, my practice began to attract more and more chronically ill patients who had been unable to get help from conventional physicians. Among them were a growing number of chemically sensitive people, a group that now accounts for over 50 percent of my patient load. Michelle was one of them.

Eating Clean and Green

To reduce the amount of toxins entering Michelle's body, I had her begin by cutting the dirty dozen fruits and vegetables out of her diet, along with all fish that's high in mercury. And while she was doing without spinach, potatoes, strawberries, and imported grapes—or bought organic versions of them instead—she was eating broccoli and drinking two or three cups of green tea every day, both of which helped her liver to clear chemicals from her body. She also cut out sugar and wheat. She'd thought that this would be harder than it turned out to be and that she would miss sugar the most. But it turned out to be breads that she longed for. When she cut them out, she found herself craving them, which shocked her. She said she felt like a breadaholic. Bread had been a staple of her diet for thirty-five years, but she'd never identified the craving before. This bothered her and made her even more determined to avoid wheat products.

Within a couple of weeks, Michelle was accustomed to the real taste of foods—the taste she'd been missing beneath all the sugar—and found she liked them better. As for breads, it took her a little longer to get used to the ones made without wheat, such as spelt and rice bread, and she never became a big fan of them. But what she learned with that experience is that she really didn't need the bread. The staff of life isn't all it's cracked up to be. She was simply used to eating it, and after a while she stopped missing it—most of the time. "When I go out to eat, I have to tell the waiter not to bring the bread basket, because if it's sitting right there in front of me, I will definitely eat a piece or three," she said.

I also had Michelle start on colonic irrigations (the importance of which I'll discuss in chapter 5), eat more fiber, and take herb supplements. Over the next three months, the pounds that had been plaguing her for decades began to disappear. The symptoms of her chemical reactivity also began to subside, including her intense allergic reactions. By the end of six months, Michelle was 20 pounds lighter and practically ecstatic. "If you'd told me it would be this easy, I never would have believed you," she said.

By the time Michelle had been living clean and green for a year, I barely recognized her. All of her symptoms were gone and her weight was down to 177 and still steadily dropping. In addition to looking and feeling better, she'd made a major decision to pursue a career path that she'd put on hold decades before. She was going back to college to get her degree in wildlife management so she could work in animal conservation. It was as if she were twenty years old again, full of energy and excitement about being alive. It was a beautiful thing to see, and something I've had the privilege of witnessing with other patients over the years.

The Art of Eating

Toxins are able to make their way into your mitochondria through the toxic foods you eat. As Michelle made very clear, cleaning up the way you eat goes a long way toward ridding your body of harmful toxins, and this will renew your energy, eliminate health problems, and free you of your excess weight. Delicious, mouthwatering foods are among life's greatest pleasures. And when you choose clean foods, you feed the powerhouses that fuel your weight loss and every vital system in your body.

Though I'm going to discuss what to eat and what not to eat to keep your diet clean, this isn't a diet, at least not in the traditional sense of counting calories (or fat grams or carbs) and obsessing over everything that goes into your mouth. This is an "I love my body" lifestyle change. Clean up your diet and you won't have to cut anything out (unless you're specifically reactive, or allergic, to certain foods), although eliminating a few specific foods would speed up the process considerably. Follow these guidelines to the art of eating and you'll lose weight and keep it off—there will be no yo-yo effect. Make these simple changes a part of your life's routine and you'll be losing weight without having to think about it.

Choose Clean Foods

I could have titled this section Eat Whole Foods or Eat Real Foods. So much of what we put into our mouths when we're hungry is more chemical than food. Soft drinks, artificial whipped cream, and processed cheese foods aren't real foods. When I was in college, a natural-foods advocate told me to steer my cart clear of the inside aisles of grocery stores and shop only on the periphery, where the produce and meat selections are. These are real foods, and when you buy the organic varieties, you're taking home far fewer chemicals. I began following her advice in my shopping and also cut out refined sugars at her insistence. I soon noticed I had an extra two hours of good energy a day—not to mention smaller grocery bills.

For centuries, our bodies ran perfectly well on clean, real, whole foods, and now we expect them to keep working well when we feed them chemicals. It's puzzling, to say the least. We know that if we put lousy gas into our cars, they won't run as well. Our bodies are no different. Think about how the first humans ate. They ate what nature provided when nature provided it. And this was exactly what they needed to nourish their cells. No shopping in the inside aisles of the grocery store for them. Our resilient bodies have managed to survive all of the bad eating habits we've since picked up, and it might sound silly to consider going back to eating like our ancient ancestors did, but the concept really isn't such a stretch. If it isn't natural, don't eat it. Easier said than done in this age of convenience, I know, but something at least worth shooting for.

The Most Important Organic Foods to Get

The cost of food—and living—is rising quickly in the United States. At one point, a gallon of gas and a gallon of milk were running neck and neck, and organic products can turn the screws even tighter. So sometimes even the most well-intentioned of us have to make tough choices when it comes time to shell out for what we eat. But remember nonorganic foods' hidden costs to you and to the world you live in. Are toxins from nonorganic foods causing the health problems that are making your days difficult? Are you going to have to spend more on health care than you saved on buying nonorganic produce?

Produce

Buy organic when you can, and always if you want one of the dirty dozen fruits and vegetables. If there are some you can't get organic, skip them altogether. It's that simple. Otherwise, stick to the clean dozen.

And when possible, buy local organic. If your organic blueberries are being shipped across the country to you, a whole lot of diesel exhaust is spewing into the air along the way. To find community-supported agriculture near you, check the resource section.

Meat

Pesticides and other toxins bioaccumulate in animals we use for food, including poultry. (Toxins are doing the same in your body, accumulating over time, reaching levels higher than in the surrounding environment.) So if you reduce your intake of meat (which will also save you money), you'll reduce your exposure to fat-soluble toxins as well. I should also mention that over the past several decades, hundreds of studies on the association between diet and health have shown overwhelmingly that people who eat the least amount of meat have the fewest chronic health problems.

Eggs and Dairy Products

Pesticides and other toxins, including DDT and PCBs, find their way into the soil and then move into grass grown in the soil, then into the cow eating the grass, then into the cow's milk—and right into you when you drink it. The process works more or less the same way with chickens and eggs.

If you're not tapped out yet and still have some items left on your shopping list, consider going as organic as you can afford. Every organic purchase you make helps your health and the planet's. You're voting with your pocketbook for a food-production system that's healthier all the way around. Remember, just 1 percent of pesticides make it to the intended pest. The other 99 percent is just out there. The success and rapid expansion of organic farming proves there's a better way.

Which Fish Is Which?

One fish, two fish, bad fish, good fish. Sounds simple, but which is which? Which kind of fish is healthy to eat and which isn't? Eating the right type of fish—tilapia over tuna, for example—makes the difference between a healthy meal and a hefty side order of mercury, PCBs, and other persistent pollutants. Farmed Atlantic salmon is just about the most toxic food you can eat today.

The United States Food and Drug Administration (FDA) has gone to the trouble of testing pretty much all the commonly available fish and seafood for mercury levels, and while I'm sure the FDA has its own larger reasons, the results also serve as a handy consumer guide. Next time you're at the seafood counter, check the list that follows for the twenty fish and seafood to steer clear of—and the twenty best bets (amounts are in parts per million). For full results, including exact mercury levels, see www.cfsan.fda.gov/%7Efrf/sea-mehg.html.

THE FDA'S TOP TWENTY BEST AND WORST MERCURY-CONTAINING FISH

Most Hg Toxic	Amount	Least Hg Toxic	Amount
Tilefish (Gulf of Mexico)	1.45	Clam	ND
Shark	0.988	Ocean perch	ND
Swordfish	0.976	Alaskan salmon (canned)	ND
King mackerel	0.730	Shrimp	ND
Bigeye tuna (fresh or frozen)	0.639	Whiting	ND
Orange roughy	0.554	Tilapia	0.010
Marlin	0.485	Oyster	0.013
Grouper	0.465	Alaskan salmon (fresh or frozen)	0.014
Mackerel, Spanish	0.454	Hake	0.014
Tuna (fresh or frozen)	0.414	Sardine	0.016
Chilean bass	0.386	Haddock	0.031
Bluefish	0.337	Crawfish	0.033
Lobster	0.310	Pollock	0.041
Croaker, white	0.287	Anchovies	0.043
Scorpion fish	0.286	Herring	0.044
Weakfish (sea trout)	0.256	Flounder or sole	0.045
Halibut	0.252	Mullet	0.046
Sablefish	0.222	Catfish	0.049
Bass (saltwater)	0.219	Scallop	0.050
Snapper	0.189	Atlantic mackerel	0.050

As you can see, the list of the most mercury-toxic fish contains some of the most commonly available fish. You'll find them at the fish counter at your grocery store, and they account for the majority of fish listed on restaurant menus. So it's safe to say that exposure to methylmercury—the form of mercury we get from fish—is very common in this country. The list of least-toxic fish, meanwhile, doesn't contain as many fish that are commonly available at restaurants and grocery stores, so you may have to make an extra stop at a fish market or an ethnic grocery store. But they're out there. And it doesn't hurt to ask whether you can special-order them.

How to Know Whether It Is Farmed Salmon

Almost all of the salmon that's farmed is Atlantic salmon, and all commercially available Atlantic salmon is farmed. There's only one species of Atlantic salmon (*Salmo salar*), and there are five Pacific salmons that belong to a genus (*Onchorhynchus*) different from Atlantic salmon. The most commonly consumed Pacific salmons include sockeye, or red, salmon (*O. nerka*), king, or chinook, salmon (*O. tshawytscha*), and silver, or coho, salmon (*O. kisutch*).

Unfortunately, because wild Pacific salmon (most of which comes from Alaska and British Columbia) costs more, some restaurants have misrepresented their farmed salmon as wild-caught Pacific fish. *The New York Times* has reported finding mislabeled fish in restaurants and fish markets alike.

Here are the ways to tell the difference:
- If the fish is labeled Salmon, it's farmed.
- If the fish is labeled Atlantic salmon, it's farmed.
- If the fish is labeled Wild salmon or if you aren't sure, ask whether it's Alaskan salmon or Atlantic. If you're told that it's Alaskan (which is Pacific salmon), ask which kind it is (red, silver, or king). If it cannot be identified as one of those three, it's farmed Atlantic.

Get Plenty of Lean Protein

Include protein with every meal. Protein is very important because it helps the liver handle the chemicals it's faced with. When your diet is low in protein, your liver is less able to break down toxic chemicals and drugs. Protein deficiency hinders all of the three components that are needed for proper phase 1 function of the liver, that crucial process that breaks down parent compounds such as alcohol in the bloodstream. Protein deficiency also impairs the liver's ability to clear toxins from the body. Besides simply staying longer in your bloodstream in their original forms, these chemicals actually become more toxic with protein deficiency. The toxicity of pesticides, herbicides, and fungicides, for example, has been shown to increase several-fold as a result of protein deficiency—as if they weren't already toxic enough.

Low-protein diets also hurt the immune system, making it more vulnerable to pesticides' toxic effects. Studies of mice showed that their ability to fight off infections and to produce antibodies to keep infections from coming back both suffered when a shortage of dietary protein opened the door to intensified DDT effects. Emotional stress was shown to have the same results. When animals were stressed, their immune systems were damaged by small levels of DDT that didn't cause the same effect in unstressed animals.

The type of protein you eat is also important. You need complete protein, even if you choose a vegetarian diet. In a study of Asian vegetarians whose diets didn't include complete proteins, chemicals remained in their bloodstreams much longer than normal because their livers couldn't flush them out efficiently. Understandably, this finding caused a lot of concern, so a group of vegetarians who consumed adequate protein were then studied. They mixed their foods properly to ensure a complete mix of essential amino acids, and it turned out that their livers worked normally.

The standard American diet—we naturopathic physicians refer to it as just plain SAD—is high in carbohydrates (sugars) and fats and low in protein. With that kind of ratio, it's hard to clear chemicals out of the bloodstream with any kind of efficiency. They're stuck in circulation for much longer than they are for people eating a more balanced diet. But for such a big problem, there's a surprisingly easy fix: eat more protein and less sugar and fat. That makes the liver function better. This kind of diet also helps with estrogen metabolism and testosterone metabolism, helping to produce the kinds of metabolites that protect against breast cancer and prostate cancer rather than promote them.

Finally, a diet high in protein interferes with the body's ability to digest and absorb fat—which is a good thing. Protein inhibits the functioning of the pancreatic enzyme known as lipase in the small intestine, which breaks fat down for absorption. But if it can't be broken down for absorption—voila—no absorption. This will be explained more fully in the next chapter.

Eat Foods That Battle Toxins

In addition to the foods we've discussed, it's wise to focus on those that will protect you from toxic damage, help your liver to properly handle toxic chemicals, and help you to move them out of your body. As amazing as it sounds, you can clear your body of toxins, prevent or reverse the damage those toxins can do, and prevent illness—and weight gain—just by eating certain foods. Let's start with foods that help undo the damage caused by toxins.

Berries

In addition to these healing oils, the compounds in berries that give them their luscious colors are also very healing. These compounds, polyphenols, are very powerful antioxidants. One of the main polyphenols, anthocyanidin, is found in very high levels in blackberries. When measured against blueberries, raspberries, red currants, and both cultivated and wild strawberries, blackberries showed the greatest antioxidant capacity. The next most potent berry is red currant, followed by raspberry, and interestingly enough, black olive was very close in power to raspberries. Similar results were found in a Norwegian study and a U.S. study. Even better, in the U.S. study, blackberries had the most antioxidant power against some of the most powerful oxidative molecules, including hydrogen peroxide. As an interesting side note, blackberries' antioxidant strength differs according to how ripe the berries are; it's strongest when they're green.

What's the big deal about antioxidants anyway? Basically, they prevent oxidative damage to tissues. The free radicals in your body—oxygen or hydrogen molecules that are unbalanced (typically missing a hydrogen atom)—steal from other molecules to make themselves complete. That's oxidation. And oxidation can disrupt the cells' normal processes. That's oxidative damage. The theft of those other electrons is like pulling the leg off a chair. The tissue is no longer balanced or complete. Most of the bodily changes we associate with aging are a result of oxidative damage—cataracts, macular degeneration, dementia, atherosclerosis, and wrinkled skin.

All of the environmental toxins cause oxidative damage, as do rancid and oxidized fats and sugars in our diets. The fat in nuts that have been stored for too long or not stored properly can become rancid. Fats can also oxidize if they become too warm for too long, which is what causes rancid butter. And when you eat these oxidized fats, you sustain oxidative damage yourself.

Heart disease, for example, occurs when one form of cholesterol (LDL) becomes oxidized, or unstable. This unstable LDL cholesterol can then damage the lining of the arteries by robbing it of those balancing electrons. Think of oxidative damage as a lighted cigarette touching something—it damages it. And this area of damage is then likely to become the site of plaque buildup that will result in plugging, or hardening, of the arteries.

Antioxidants prevent or slow free radicals' theft of electrons. Besides berry pigments, antioxidants include vitamins C and E, beta-carotene, and other natural compounds, all of which serve to extinguish the cigarette or replace the leg on the chair. They also prevent the leg from sustaining further damage. So the higher the level of antioxidants in our bodies, the lower the level of tissue damage.

In chapter 1 I talked a lot about mitochondria and the serious damage that environmental chemicals can do to these all-important energy factories inside each of our cells. While all antioxidants help to protect our mitochondria, one study has shown blackberry juice to have the ability to reverse the suppression of mitochondrial function caused by potent free radicals known as peroxynitrites and prevent them from damaging blood vessels. This has huge implications for the prevention of stroke, heart attacks, and chronic neurological problems such as Parkinson's and Alzheimer's, as these particular free radicals have been clearly linked to such problems. The ability to quench peroxynitrites also makes this a very valuable defensive weapon for anyone taking the amino acid L-arginine or any of the Viagra-type products. All of those compounds increase the production of nitric oxide in the body, which ultimately breaks down to peroxynitrites. So, men who wish to preserve their brains along with their erections should be consuming a lot of berries or berry extracts every day.

Besides being found in blackberries, these wonderful polyphenols known as anthocyanidins can also be found in blueberries, and frozen blueberries are available in grocery stores year-round. The benefit of using frozen berries is that the freezing breaks down the cell walls, so the berry pigments are even more available to us than when the berries are fresh. A half-cup of frozen berries a day is an excellent addition to your diet.

Green Tea and Broccoli

When it comes to helping the liver properly process chemicals in the blood, the two most powerful foods are green tea and broccoli (and its brassica cousins: cauliflower, brussels sprouts, cabbage, and kale). Broccoli boosts the enzymes that help move caffeine and some airborne pollutants out of our blood, and it boosts glutathione function, which helps usher out toxins such as pesticides and solvents. Eat broccoli raw or juiced for peak benefits, or use broccoli sprouts on your salad—they have the highest levels of these beneficial chemicals. Beyond broccoli and other brassicas, great choices with similar properties are beets and liberal amounts of turmeric, ginger, and rosemary.

As for green tea, it works wonders on several fronts. Among them, it helps your body release fat from storage, supports the liver in its mission to clear toxins from the blood, and helps fat-soluble toxins leave the body with your stool. Yes, green tea helps usher toxins all the way from their storage space in your fat tissue to the toilet. No other natural compound has such profound power over these toxins that are so reluctant to leave our bodies. This ability may be one reason that green tea use has been associated with reduced rates of cancer, but green tea also appears to hurry cancer cells along to the self-destruction that awaits aged cells. Drinking green tea on a regular basis reduces the risk of stomach cancer by 48 percent and cuts the risk of chronic gastritis (inflammation of the stomach) by 51 percent, according to a study done in China, where stomach cancer rates are high.

Meanwhile, another study in China showed that green tea is tremendously beneficial in the prevention of ovarian cancer. Daily green tea drinkers had a 61 percent lower risk of developing this form of cancer than those who didn't drink green tea. Those who drank it every day for more than thirty years had an even greater reduction in risk (76 percent less). So, the more green tea you drink every day and the longer you drink it, the better it works.

Green tea has also been shown to be effective in preventing the development of full-blown prostate tumors in men. When thirty men diagnosed with the presence of prostate cancer cells were given 600 milligrams of catechins—the active health agents found in green tea—every day for a year (roughly the equivalent of 4 cups a day), only one man had developed a tumor by the end of a year, while 30 percent of the control group did. With prostate cancer as common as it is, I can't think of a single reason that men concerned about their prostates shouldn't be drinking green tea or taking a green tea extract every day. And yes, I practice what I preach.

Many of the people I've talked to about green tea, including Michelle, have told me they don't like the taste of it. I felt the same way when I started drinking it, and now I love it. It's amazing how your taste buds can adjust to accommodate what your body knows is good for it—try it. And Michelle will back me up on this. She didn't like broccoli either, but she's learned to. And she tells me it just wouldn't be the same if she didn't wash it down with some green tea.

A number of tea flavors are available now. If, like me, you can't stand the green tea mixed with toasted rice, try jasmine green tea—when it's good, it's great. If you look in the tea aisle of the grocery store, you'll find a surprisingly diverse selection to choose from. Republic of Tea has many wonderful flavors, and I drink a lot of the Safeway O Organics green tea. My wife's favorite is the green iced tea from Starbucks.

Green tea is also beneficial for our mental functioning, providing powerful brain protection. People who drink two or more cups of green tea a day are 54 percent less likely to experience the typical cognitive decline that happens as we age. And those who drink a cup a day are 38 percent less likely to develop dementia. So, with daily green tea intake, the loss of mental function doesn't have to be a part of the aging process. Not only do the polyphenols in green tea pass through the blood-brain barrier and serve as protective anti-oxidants for the precious brain cells (neurons), but they can also chelate iron from them (chelation is a process by which molecules can grab heavy metals and move them out of the body). This prevents iron buildup inside the neurons, a condition that promotes oxidative damage and is associated with the development of parkinsonism and other chronic neurologic diseases. In animal models, green tea blocks the neurotoxin MPTP's ability to induce Parkinson's, which is truly astounding, because exposure to MPTP can lead to the development of Parkinson's-like symptoms within hours. That's akin to stopping a speeding bullet. Fortunately, MPTP isn't a common chemical in our environment—it's actually a contaminant in synthetic heroin—but it's nice to know green tea can fight off something so powerful.

Among green tea's other benefits:

- It's been shown to have an antianxiety effect in animal studies. The effect is similar to what happened when psychoactive drugs (benzodiazepines) were administered to the animals.
- It provides protection for the heart.
- People who drink green tea daily (more than two cups) are about 30 percent less likely to die from cardiovascular disease than those who don't. The biggest protection is against the risk of dying from stroke.

According to two studies, drinking a couple of cups of green tea a day significantly increases levels of normal healthy intestinal bacteria and decreases levels of disease-causing bacteria and fecal odor. The bacteria in our bowels contribute greatly to our overall immune functioning and our ability to process waste, clear toxins from our bowels, and maintain proper digestion and absorption. Probiotics are supplements available at health food stores that contain one or more of these healthy bacteria. With regular use, they can help to repopulate the bowels with the bacteria that should be there. Tea drinkers in the studies experienced greatly increased levels of both of the healthy bowel bacteria—bifidobacteria and lactobacilli—and reduced levels of the unhealthy bacteria—Bacteroidaceae, Enterobacteriaceae, and clostridia. They also enjoyed a reduction in the compounds in their stool that cause bad odor, including ammonia, indole, and skatole. And this healthy rebalancing of the bowel flora occurred only with green tea—there was no need to take probiotics.

When it comes to green tea, there's something to be said for heavy drinking. Consuming ten or more cups a day has been shown to prevent chronic atrophic gastritis (a problem found in more than 80 percent of people over the age of sixty-five), even when those people have inflammation-causing *H. pylori* infections. Also, the risk of green tea drinkers developing chronic gastritis is 51 percent lower than it is for those who don't drink green tea, and the risk of developing stomach cancer is also cut in half. And the more they drank and the longer they'd been drinking green tea, the higher their risk reduction for both problems.

All of these formidable benefits make green tea one of the most powerful bonus nutrients in existence. Other foods that help enhance the excretion of toxins from the body include dark green leafy vegetables, seaweeds, rice bran, and brown rice. The more of these you eat, the more toxins you'll be escorting out of your body.

Eat Good, Clean Fat Only—and Not Too Much

Be careful about the fat you eat (what kind and how much), because most toxins are stored in fat. That is, besides being stored in the fat in your body, they may be stored in whatever fat you ingest—butter, for example, or that beautifully marbled steak you had the other night. But this isn't a rigid no-fat diet. Fats are actually necessary to be healthy. As mentioned before, some fats are absolutely essential for the proper functioning of the body yet can't be manufactured in the body. These are called essential fatty acids or essential fats, and they include the omega-3 and omega-6 oils found in fish and certain vegetables and seeds. But before I get into the specific benefits of omega-3 and omega-6 oils, let's take a commercial break.

Do you want lustrous hair (the kind advertisements say you can get only with certain types of hair products)? Do you want healthy skin (the kind advertisements say you can get only with certain skin lotions)? Do you want to sleep through the night without having to wake up to eat? Do you want a brain that works well and nerves that don't "short out"? Do you want all of the chemical messages in your body to make it to the intended cells? If so, add some fat to your diet!

In all seriousness, fats provide all of these benefits and more. They're necessary for the health of our skin, our mucus membranes, and our hair. They provide the fuel our bodies run on when we go without eating overnight. They provide the insulation surrounding our nerves and function as the "windows" into each cell through which messages come and go.

But different types of fats have different types of effects in the body on a biochemical level. The biggest area of impact is in the level of inflammation. Our bodies use some of the fat we consume to produce chemical compounds called prostaglandins; some prostaglandins cause inflammation, and some reduce inflammation (they're natural anti-inflammatories, kind of like your own ibuprofen factory). Saturated fats—fats that are solid at room temperature, such as cheese, butter, and beef fat—crank up production of inflammation-causing prosta-glandins. But when you consume the essential fatty acids omega-3 and omega-6 oils (all are liquid at room temperature) in the form of fish, flax, and safflower oils, you shift your prostaglandin production to the anti-inflammatory side.

Fish Oil

In my naturopathic practice, I regularly recommend that patients take fish oil capsules in addition to eating nontoxic fish regularly. I've seen people who are in pain and use ibuprofen on a daily basis finally get rid of the pain when they start taking several capsules of fish oil a day. Many of these people also show up with dry skin (especially on their lower legs) and report that they use moisturizers every day. Not only will their inflammation improve by taking fish oil capsules, but so will their skin.

Fish oil contains two main oils, eicosapentaenoic acid (EPA) and docosahexaenoic acid (DHA), and has been documented to improve the brain power of children whose mothers ate fish regularly during pregnancy and breastfeeding. Parents of children with ADHD often report that their children's conditions improve when taking fish oil or just the DHA. Japanese research has shown that DHA suppresses free radicals in the brain that are caused by exposure to organophosphate pesticides. This powerful brain protection may be the reason DHA enhances IQ in children and benefits memory.

I still remember James, a patient who came to me when he was in his mid-fifties. One of his main complaints was diminished brain power, but I also noted that the skin on his lower legs was so dry that it was almost shiny. One of the supplements I recommended for him was DHA. When he came back six weeks later and I asked him how the supplement regimen was going, he was so excited he almost flew out of the chair. While he was happy with all of them, saying they were all doing what they were supposed to, he positively raved about the DHA. He said, "It gave me my brain back." He'd thought that the fading brain power was just a factor of getting older and that all he could do about it was make "senior jokes"—in other words, just grin and bear it. But his brain was in fine shape; it just needed the right oils to keep it functioning as it should. And James wasn't an unusual case—proper nutrition and supplementation can make a huge difference for most of us.

Olive Oil

Besides making sure you're getting enough of the essential oils, make sure the oils you're using aren't rancid. Antioxidants are added to most oils to head off rancidity if they don't contain natural antioxidants. And most olive oils come in dark bottles to cut down on the light that makes it through to the oil, which can cause it to become rancid. But most of the rancid oils we consume come from almonds and other nuts that have been around for too long. If they leave a rancid taste in your mouth, pitch them—ingesting rancid oils causes significant oxidative damage in the body.

Speaking of olive oil, while it isn't considered an essential oil, it is a very healthy oil. Researchers who have studied the high–olive oil diet in Mediterranean countries have repeatedly shown that this high-fat diet helps prevent heart disease. Women with diets higher in olive oil have also been shown to have lower rates of breast cancers. So choose your oils wisely and use the healthy ones liberally in your diet.

Eliminate Trans Fats

In addition to the pesticides, plastics, heavy metals, and combustion byproducts that lurk in food, awaiting their chance to poison your mitochondria and cause fatigue, some energy-sapping compounds are added to foods intentionally. Trans fats, for example, are in lots of processed foods and made the news recently when McDonald's and other restaurants stopped using them. Research showing the adverse effects of these compounds has been around for a while, but recent studies on mitochondrial function also show a startling connection. When rats were fed a diet high in trans fats (similar to what someone who eats a lot of junk food consumes), their level of mitochondrial function dropped by 13 percent. These trans fats start life as real fats that are liquid at room temperature, but they're put through a process that changes their structure so that they become solid at room temperature. Originally, it was thought that trans fats would be good for the diet because they don't elevate cholesterol levels. But it turns out that the body just doesn't know what to do with them. They can't be burned for fuel, and research shows that when they're transported to the mitochondria to be used as fuel, they throw a wrench into the works and interfere with their function.

Eat Less Refined Sugar

You're no doubt already familiar with some of the problematic aspects of sugar—the calories, the crash—but for our purposes, the key point is that sugar hinders the liver's ability to clear toxic compounds from the bloodstream. This was discovered in 1951 when researchers tested two groups of rats: one group was given phenobarbital intravenously and the other group was given glucose as well as phenobarbital. The rats were sedated because of the phenobarbital, but those given glucose remained sedated longer than those that weren't. This was a clear sign that an elevated sugar level in the blood prevented the liver from doing its job efficiently. And further research revealed that like protein deficiency, sugar obstructs components we need for proper functioning of the phase 1 pathway in the liver. A high-sugar diet also impairs one of the primary detoxification functions of the liver.

Meanwhile in a study of humans, a group of volunteers ate a high-carb diet for two weeks, then a high-fat diet for two weeks, and finally a high-protein diet for two weeks. They were also given the medications antipyrine and theophylline, and their ability to clear these compounds from the blood was monitored throughout the six weeks. During the high-carb and high-fat weeks, the chemicals remained in their bloodstreams for much longer than they did during the high-protein weeks. And for the record, the numbers of calories consumed were consistent throughout the six weeks, so it wasn't a caloric discrepancy that caused the difference—it was the types of calories. The lesson is that by simply substituting some dietary protein for either carbs or fats in your food choices, your liver will do a much better job of kicking out the chemicals that shouldn't be loitering in your bloodstream. It's a small sacrifice with a big payoff.

Even people with liver problems can benefit. When we discussed yo-yo dieting, I mentioned that those dieters can end up developing fatty liver disease (also called hepatic steatosis). This problem is associated with diabetes and can lead to the development of more severe liver disease. When eleven patients with this nasty problem who were eating high-sugar diets were studied, their liver cells were initially dying at an unhealthy rate, and the clearance of chemicals from their blood was compromised. After eating a sugar-restricted diet for two months, their chemical-clearance abilities recovered and the rate at which their liver cells were dying slowed to a normal rate. Good thing, because they need those cells.

If you really want to make a difference, cut out sugars altogether. This is especially true if you're a sugar addict—which you are if you can't make it through the day without sugar. Sugar is one of the three most reactive foods—most likely to trigger what some people refer to as food allergies—along with wheat and dairy products. If we'd all stop eating sugar and wheat products, a huge improvement in health problems would sweep the nation. In the United States, we're averaging 2 to 3 pounds of sugar per person a week! And we've gone from consuming 45 pounds of high-fructose corn syrup a year to consuming 66 pounds a year since 1985. What's really scary is that some of us don't consume that much—like me—and there are people out there who are picking up our slack. Over the past century, the percentage of calories from sugar in Americans' diet rose from 13 percent to 20 percent. That means that more than half of our daily calories come from some form of sugar, factoring in carbohydrates' 40 percent chunk of our diet. No wonder sugar is causing so many health problems. It's been known for years that when you consume something that boosts your blood sugar, the vitamin C level in your white blood cells (your infection-fighters) drops by 50 percent and remains depressed for about five hours. The white cells' ability to eat invading bacteria and viruses is also depressed by 50 percent for that five-hour period. Haven't you noticed that kids often get sick after Halloween, Easter, and other high-sugar times?

In addition to suppressing your immune function, causing fatigue, and increasing the risk of diabetes (and therefore heart disease), sugar intake may have something to do with cancer rates. In a study done in Seattle about twenty years ago on dietary sugars' impact on the development of breast cancer in rodents, the rodents were injected with a set number of breast-cancer cells and fed one of three diets: low-sugar, regular-sugar, and high-sugar. Of those in the regular-sugar diet (whose blood sugar averaged 100 milligrams per deciliter), 50 percent died from cancer at the end of the month, while 75 percent of those on the high-sugar, diet (with an average blood sugar level of 120 milligrams per deciliter) died. But only one mouse (0.5 percent) in the low-sugar group (with an average blood sugar of 80 milligrams per deciliter) succumbed. This could very well indicate that consuming the amount of sugar that Americans do could affect our bodies' ability to fight cancer.

Do you need any more incentive to cut out refined sugar? If so, how about this: honey. It's delicious and natural. But since a teaspoon of it is twice as sweet as the same amount of white sugar, use just a little to sweeten what you're eating or drinking. Isn't it good to know that with things like dates and figs also up her sleeve—and all other manner of fruit—Mother Nature didn't neglect our sweet tooth?

These guidelines for the art of eating are the foundation for clean, healthy eating. Once you've followed them for a few weeks, you'll realize how easy it is to eat this way. And for at least the first four weeks, put away your scale and focus on how you feel. The toxins will begin leaving your body immediately, but it can take up to six weeks for your toxic load to drop low enough for the weight to start to come off. But it will come off, and you'll start to feel better.

If you want faster results, however, and you're ready to make more of a commitment to changing how you eat, there are a few other changes I recommend. While the foods that follow aren't on the most-toxic list, the reactions they cause in the body become part of your total toxic burden. Cutting them out of your diet is a key to rapid results and a sure way to feel better. Are you ready for the first change? You may have to sit down for this one: stop eating wheat.

Kick Your Daily Bread Habit

Although whole wheat breads, pastas, and cereals are touted as much healthier than products made from white flour—which is essentially bleached, refined wheat—they're all made from wheat. And besides being one of the most commonly reactive foods, wheat contains a protein—gluten—that many people can't tolerate. When they eliminate these two types of reactivity from their lives, most people feel much better.

Many of the nagging symptoms that plague people in their daily lives can be traced back to what is essentially an overdose of this one food that the body is trying to reject. The common symptoms that people with adverse reactions to wheat experience include headaches, fatigue, mood swings, depression, inability to lose weight, eczema, chronic sinus problems, allergies, and arthritis. I can't count the times that patients have said they feel decades younger a couple of months after I'd asked them to ban wheat from their diets.

How can you tell whether wheat is a potential problem for you? Well, first of all, do you have any of the problems I just listed? If so, you're likely to be reactive to wheat (either whole wheat or white flour products). Next, how often do you eat wheat-containing products? If you eat them three times a week or more, the wheat may be causing your problems. If you eat them every day, it's much more likely to cause health problems. Finally, if you find yourself craving it, there's no doubt—you are reactive to wheat.

So, what can you do about it? Take a look at all of the foods in your diet with an eye toward uncovering the hidden sources of wheat, typically listed on the label as flour. It's found in most breads and is also present in many soups, gravies, and even soy sauce. An easy way to avoid wheat is to shop for gluten-free baked goods and pastas. For more details on leading a gluten-free life, see the four-week plan in chapter 7 and the resource section. Information on how to get tested for adverse food reactions is also available in the resource section.

Refined wheat is a simple carbohydrate that immediately breaks down into sugar in the body and raises blood sugar very quickly. Eliminate wheat from your diet—and get rid of all sugar—and you'll start to lose weight almost immediately. And remember breada-holic Michelle's experience: kicking the habit was easier than she'd expected.

Got Milk? Too Bad

Dairy is the other most common reactive food, and people who don't see enough improvement after cutting out wheat and sugar should try taking dairy out of their diets, too. If you react to wheat, sugar, and dairy and you stop eating just one of these foods, you may not notice much improvement—you need to cut out all three of these foods to feel better. My patients who stop eating all three foods tell me they feel like entirely new people. Ron, for example, was in his late sixties and working at a local car dealership when I helped him to change his life. He reported that he'd been active and healthy until he injured his knee while playing golf a few years before.

"Then everything went downhill," he said. "My body feels old, but my brain still thinks I'm young."

He was grossly overweight and had elevated blood pressure, diabetes, and autoimmune arthritis in his hand joints. Tired of just being handed pharmaceutical drugs to take, he was convinced there was a better way.

By now, I'm sure it will come as no surprise to you that there was a better way. First I prescribed a diet free of sugar, wheat, and dairy. Ron had been starting each day with an English muffin and a latte (with milk), and eating a lot of pasta with cheese at dinner. But his new diet was an entirely different story. Thanks to the increasing public awareness of gluten sensitivity, he was able to find great gluten-free English muffins at his local grocery store. He began using rice or soy milk in place of cow's milk and switched to goat cheese and soy cheese while he was at it. He even found some local restaurants that offer gluten-free menus, so he didn't feel deprived of the opportunity to treat himself by dining out. And for his pasta fix, he found that the grocery store also had rice pasta for him to cook at home, which he ended up loving.

The first couple of weeks were a little frustrating for Ron, with a fair amount of trial and error, but then he found that he was able to completely avoid the problem foods without much trouble. For his lunches out, for instance, he just needed to think ahead when choosing a restaurant. And he found that he was just as satisfied eating salads as he had been with sandwiches.

Then I tested Ron for heavy-metal burden. It wasn't surprising to find that he had an elevated lead level, since I often find heavy-metal burden in people with high blood pressure. He started taking oral chelators to eliminate the lead and a supplement protocol outlined in chapter 5.

By his six-week follow-up, Ron's blood pressure had dropped 10 points, his weight was down by 5 pounds, and his blood sugar had dropped. But the biggest changes he reported were his renewed energy and his general feeling of wellness. His mood had improved with his energy, and he said he felt better than he had in a long time.

Ron continued on the supplement protocol for eighteen months, during which we had regular visits so I could keep tabs on him, and the end result was that he felt—and looked—like a new, much younger man.

CHAPTER 4

Out with the Bad

Victoria came to see me when she was in her mid-sixties and very overweight. She'd started putting on the pounds while going through menopause, and it built from there. In the last year alone, she'd gained 20 pounds. She was working with a personal trainer at a gym twice a week and closely watching her diet, but the number on the scale kept climbing. Needless to say, she was frustrated and dejected because she wasn't getting anywhere. Unfortunately, this is a common occurrence for many people. They do the best they can and take the steps that are conventionally thought to be the most effective, but they don't get the results they're looking for.

Victoria's health history—which included chronic constipation—was the very picture of toxicity. It had been so many years since she was regular—having one to three bowel movements a day—that she thought that going just three or four times a week was normal. Even if she hadn't been constipated, her toxic load would have been high, but having a slow and sluggish elimination system was making matters worse. Day by day, she was getting heavier and becoming more toxic.

Victoria had autoimmune arthritis that was so severe she couldn't even pick up her one-year-old grandson (the one person who put a smile on her face every day). She said her thinking had been muddled lately and she was worried she might be getting Alzheimer's disease. She had lymphoma (which until recently had been in remission for four years) and chemical sensitivity. And tests showed that she had elevated mercury levels and an extremely high lead level. The mercury had most likely come from the fish she ate and her amalgam dental fillings. The lead was another story: about 95 percent of lead is stored in bones, and when bone loss starts with menopause, lead is released into the body. And sure enough, Victoria traced the origins of almost all of her health issues—the arthritis, the high blood pressure, the brain fog, the weight gain—back to the time when she was going through menopause. This is why the change of life is such a critical time for women to be proactive. A woman approaching the cessation of her menses should be talking to a licensed naturopathic physician about the steps she needs to take to be optimally healthy.

Victoria began following the guidelines for the art of eating and put her house on a "diet" (the steps for which I'll cover in chapter 7). One of the most important things for her to do was to significantly increase the amount of fiber in her diet and the amount of water she was drinking. She also needed to get the nutrients that bind and remove fat-soluble toxins and that help her liver clear chemicals from her body. To mobilize lead and mercury from her body, she started an oral chelation protocol with a compound called meso-2,3-dimercaptosuccinic acid (DMSA), which is very effective at escorting these metals out of the body.

Everyone's different, but when I'm helping a patient to lower toxic burden, there tends to be an order in which we notice improvements. Usually energy and the brain are the first to improve, and that's precisely what happened for Victoria. Within just a few weeks, she was having a bowel movement every day, she had more mental clarity and lower blood pressure, and she said she didn't feel quite as tired. The production of energy and the working of the brain cells depend a lot on what's circulating in the bloodstream, so eliminating toxins floating around in there can lead to a rapid change that's easily noticeable. It can take a longer time to see improvements in other organs and

Oral Chelation Supplements

While a number of oral supplements are touted as having the ability to clear heavy metals from the body, only three of them have been scientifically validated. Two of the following compounds are available only by prescription through a physician, and for good reason. These compounds need to be used as part
of a complete heavy-metal reduction protocol. They should not be taken without supervision or by themselves, and the protocol should be overseen by a physician who's very familiar with supporting people who are mobilizing powerful toxins in their bodies.

- DMSA— meso-2,3-dimercaptosuccinic acid—has been thoroughly studied over the past couple of decades and is both safe and effective for the mobilization of lead and mercury. It isn't available at health food stores and should be used only under the direction of a physician trained in heavy-metal chelation.
- NAC— N-acetyl-L-cysteine—is an amino acid that is available at health food stores. It's been shown to increase the excretion of methylmercury from the body, so it's a wonderful supplement to take if you've been eating any of the mercury-containing fish. It doesn't enhance the excretion of elemental mercury from dental fillings, however.
- DMPS—sodium salt of 2,3-dimercapto-1-propane sulfonate—is a well-studied molecule that's available for either intravenous or oral use when prescribed by a physician. It's very efficient at enhancing the clearance of mercury from the body and has been documented to be both safe and effective.

None of the other so-called heavy-metal chelators on the market are backed by any research to prove that they're effective. I've tested several on patients who have a heavy-metal burden, and we saw no improvement in the clearance of heavy metals.

tissues, but I fully expected to see Victoria's weight start to drop within another few weeks. She wasn't nearly as confident about this as I was, but within two months of being clean and green, she dropped a dress size, had significantly less arthritis pain, and her chemical sensitivity tapered off. Experiencing these changes, which Victoria described as miracles, made such a profound impact on her that she easily committed to making this a way of life. And by the end of six months, without having to do anything else differently with diet or exercise, she'd lost 50 pounds.

You've already learned a little about stopping toxins from making their way into your body, but, like Victoria, you still need to get rid of what's inevitably already there. Getting rid of the toxins that are keeping you fat will automatically make you slimmer as you become cleaner and healthier. One of the ways you're going to do that is by—forgive me—pooping. As the cleansing adage goes, better out than in! The truth is that the best way to eliminate existing toxins is to *actually* eliminate them. And as your body begins to clear the toxins, your mitochondria will be restored to full power and so will you. With energy creation getting a jump-start, you'll also begin burning off fat stores in your body the old-fashioned way: by metabolizing them.

This chapter will explain the process of casting toxins out of the temple—your body. It will also cover the "wonder drug" orlistat and its natural alternatives. And for those who prefer a paragon of junk food that's been proven to enhance excretion of dioxins, PCBs, and other toxins from the human body, this chapter will cover fat-free Pringles with olestra.

You'll also find out how to increase the amount of toxins exiting your body, not just through your intestines, but also through your kidneys and your skin, and by optimizing your liver function. Finally, I'll talk about elimination of estrogens. If the process doesn't work efficiently, estrogen imbalances can lead to water retention and, as a result, weight gain.

Clearing the Main Exit

As everyone is aware, the bowel is the main pathway for waste to leave the body. Given the amount of junk we put into the opening of the gastrointestinal (GI) system, we might expect a lot to leave at the other end. Unfortunately, most people don't seem to have regular bowel movements even though they regularly put food into their mouths. It's a simple equation: if fecal matter isn't leaving the body at the same rate that food is going in, there will be a problem. The bloodstream is absorbing compounds that should be leaving the body, including toxic compounds that have a difficult enough time leaving as it is. Conventional wisdom says that if you have one bowel movement a day, you're regular, but most people eat at least three times a day. Yes, that means that ideally we'd move our bowels three times a day. And yes, it's doable. When I was in college, before I started cleansing, I was having bowel movements only about twice a week—thanks to the good old standard American diet I was eating in the cafeteria and at fast-food restaurants. After I started cleansing, I began to have daily bowel movements. As I continued to cleanse, I got to where I was having three healthy bowel movements a day. That's the goal. This way the waste products aren't sitting in your bowels and getting sucked back into the bloodstream to make you feel—ahem—crappy.

So many people have trouble with their bowels that laxative sales in the United States total over $1 billion a year. Some of this is due to our low-fiber diet, which will be helped dramatically by the changes discussed in chapter 3. Another cause is magnesium deficiency. This is one of the most commonly deficient nutrients among my patients. Severe magnesium deficiency causes hard, dry stools that often look like rabbit pellets. Other common symptoms are headaches, muscle spasms, insomnia, heart palpitations, premenstrual tension, and chocolate craving. Whenever our bodies are exposed to chemicals (including drugs and alcohol), we lose a lot of magnesium through urination, so when you consider how great our toxic burden is, it's no surprise that magnesium deficiency is so common.

Other common causes of constipation include eating foods that you're reactive or allergic to; reduced output of hydrochloric acid in your stomach, which can be caused by illness, toxic overload, and heartburn medicine; a sluggish thyroid gland; and overgrowth of *Candida albicans* yeast in your intestines, which can be caused by the use of steroids, antibiotics, and oral contraceptives. If you have a severe constipation problem, it really is worth a visit to a licensed

naturopathic physician to get it straightened out. Go to www.naturo
pathic.org to find a licensed naturopathic physician near you.

Increase the Amount of Toxins
Leaving Your Body

Once your body's main elimination system is working smoothly, it's
time to increase the amount of toxins that can leave through that
door.

Toxins build up in our bodies because they have a hard time leaving.
With the exception of the heavy metals, which account for less than 5
percent of our toxic load, they're fat-soluble compounds. Whenever
they try to leave our bodies, the natural fat-recycling mechanisms
collar them and send them back into the bloodstream. So, to reduce
the total body load of these compounds, methods that serve to guide
these toxins out of the body need to be explored.

Now that Victoria was eating clean and green foods and dumping
more toxins and more fat, I wanted to reduce her toxin load quickly
and ensure that toxins were leaving her body. When I requested that
as part of her program she start on colonic irrigations, I got the kind
of response I usually get.

"You're joking, right?" she said through her laughter.

"Madam, I never indulge in toilet humor," I assured her. "But seriously, I'd just like you to give this a shot because most of my patients
who've tried it *swear* by it. You don't want to argue with success, do
you?"

"I'm not sure," she said. "I'm not thrilled about it, but I guess I'm
willing to try it if you say it really is important."

I explained to Victoria that the reason I wanted to start her on
colonics was that I've found them to be extremely effective for all
forms of autoimmune diseases. In my practice, close to 100 percent of
my autoimmune patients who do colonic irrigations see a reversal
of their autoimmunity problems. Their symptoms go away, and their
blood levels of autoantibodies—which damage tissue—drop into normal ranges. It's a very simple procedure that rapidly reduces the level
of circulating toxins in the body. While few patients are happy with the
notion of doing colonics, what I'd told Victoria was true: after starting

them, many of my patients become downright evangelistic about them because of the health benefits they experience.

I've used colonic irrigations in my practice for more than twenty-five years to give toxins the boot. It's a simple process with no real discomfort involved; a small price to pay for a clean colon, which is the last stop in the digestion process. Specifically, the colon's job is to control the loss of water from the body while prompting fecal matter and a host of toxic compounds to leave (some of which would rather hang around). When constipation prevents the colon from carrying out this vital function, disease is a distinct possibility. As Grace Bliss, my first mentor in healthy living, used to say, "All disease starts in the colon." Over the years, I've found that Grace was largely right.

Besides colonics, current research has revealed other methods that are also effective at keeping the colon running smoothly. They work their magic more slowly than colonics, but if you have the time, they're a great option.

One of the first compounds that showed an ability to clear fat-soluble toxins from the body was the food additive olestra. Olestra is a fat you can't absorb, so during its brief stay in your body, it's confined to the intestine until eventually leaving with the rest of your food waste. Apparently, the idea for putting it in food is that it will allow us to eat foods containing the nice flavors that fats provide without gaining any weight. There's also the fact that any amount of fat in the bowels attracts fat-soluble toxins to it, so when you increase the amount of fat in the stool, you automatically increase the amount of fat-soluble toxins leaving the body. Unfortunately, excretion of the fat-soluble vitamins A, D, E, and K and the essential fatty acids (found in fish oil and some seed oils) also occurs with olestra, resulting in deficiencies. But the most compromising side effect is the infamous anal leakage, the uncontrollable loose movements we heard so much about when olestra was added to Pringles in the late nineties. This has resulted in a drastic reduction in the use of olestra in foods despite its possible benefits.

Those benefits appear to be very real. In a study of three volunteers who consumed 25 grams of olestra a day, the excretion of various fat-soluble toxins jumped to a rate that was a whopping 11 times the norm. The olestra approach was later incorporated successfully in the case of two women who were severely poisoned with 2,3,7, 8-TCDD, the most toxic of all dioxins, at their workplace.

The most illuminating case study was conducted on an overweight diabetic male in Australia who had been severely poisoned with PCBs and was afflicted with headaches, numbness, and tingling in his lower body, and the painful skin condition chloracne, a common symptom of PCB overload. Because of his short stature, he was listed as obese at only 222 pounds. He also had elevated cholesterol and was insulin dependent. Whenever he tried to lose weight, his chloracne, the numbness, and the tingling became worse, obviously because of the surge in PCB circulation that comes with fat breakdown. Based on the previously published studies, his physicians arranged for him to eat an amount of potato chips containing 16 grams of olestra a day—a level low enough to head off any of its negative side effects. After two years of eating just seven olestra-containing potato chips a day, the man had lost almost 40 pounds, his cholesterol was normal, he was no longer diabetic, and his PCB level had dropped from 1,254 milligrams per kilogram to 56. And he was able to do all of this without altering his diet in any other way and without suffering any of the side effects of weight loss he'd previously experienced.

During these two years, the olestra allowed him to clear out a little more PCBs every day through his stool than he could before, setting off a fascinating domino effect. As the overall PCB level dropped in his body, the level of PCBs taking a toll on his mitochondria naturally dropped as well. This led to an improvement in fat breakdown and thermogenesis, which dumped more PCBs into his bloodstream, which in turn were cleared out through the bowels. In short, the PCBs left the body instead of just recirculating and causing more symptoms. The icing on the cake was that as his mitochondrial function improved, his diabetes, fatigue, and obesity—all clearly associated in medical literature with mitochondrial dysfunction—got better as well.

Does this mean we all need to start taking olestra every day like we would a multivitamin? No. Fortunately, there are natural means of enhancing the excretion of fecal fat. But the results of these olestra studies show the importance of moving toxins out of the body through excretion. It's just that olestra isn't the best way to go, since it prevents those who aren't overweight from absorbing the fat-soluble vitamins they need.

Researchers have been looking for methods that don't use olestra to help clear PCBs from the body. What they've found confirms that rice bran fibers (RBF) and chlorophyll-containing compounds (green veggies) top the list of effective natural agents. Rice bran fiber is found naturally in whole-grain brown rice but isn't present in white rice (or the kind of fried rice you get at most Chinese restaurants). If you don't eat brown rice regularly, you can get brown rice fiber at your local health-food store or from a naturopathic physician.

RBF has been shown to bind easily with PCBs and other toxins, including the combustion byproduct BAP, in a laboratory setting. In animal studies, RBF has also proved capable of dramatically diminishing the reabsorption—or hepatic recycling—of PCBs from the intestines. Hepatic recycling occurs when the liver dumps some of these toxins into the intestines, where they're reabsorbed into the bloodstream and sent back to the liver. This recycling pattern is the main reason that so many toxins never make it out of the body—talk about a vicious circle.

Whereas RBF helps break this recycling pattern and force more toxins to leave, wheat bran has shown absolutely no benefit in this regard. A study using spinach fiber and RBF in animals that had been exposed to PCBs showed that RBF increased fecal PCB excretion 6.6 times, and spinach fiber increased it 4.1 times. Another animal study showed that animals eating a diet of 10 percent RBF excreted 4.5 times more highly toxic compounds than animals eating the same diet without the fiber. And in several studies of patients with Yusho disease—contracted in 1968 from cooking oil contaminated with PCBs—after they consumed 7 to 10 grams of a fermented RBF product three times a day for a year, they had twice the amount of dioxin excretion as their counterparts who consumed less fiber. This means the PCBs were beating a retreat from the body twice as fast as normal—and without the help of colonics! And by the way, yes, the effects of Yusho disease are still being felt four decades later, both by the people who consumed the PCB-laden oil and by their offspring— that's how dangerous PCBs are.

Chlorophyll, meanwhile, has long been thought of as a blood purifier, and recent studies have documented its effectiveness at helping to clear persistent chemical pollutants from the body. Both spinach fiber and matcha green tea can increase the excretion of chlorinated pollutants from the body, and both of these compounds include chlorophyll. Coincidence? Probably not. When the seaweed nori, which also contains chlorophyll, was tested on rats, the rats fed a diet that was 10 percent nori experienced increases in fecal excretion of dioxins at levels 5.5 and 6.0 times higher than the control group did. Chlorella, long a popular detoxification agent, was also tested, and the group of rats given chlorella experienced increased dioxin excretion that varied from 30 percent to more than 300 percent higher than the control group's. Hypothesizing that the chlorophyll was responsible for the results, the researchers then fed the rats diets with chlorophyll levels ranging from 0.1 percent to 0.5 percent (that's about the same as making organic spinach 10 percent of your diet or seaweed 20 percent of your diet). In the 0.1 percent group, the fecal excretion of the various toxins ranged from 40 percent to 80 percent greater than for the control group. At the end of the study, all of the animals given the chlorophyll had lower total body burdens of these persistent toxins than their counterparts.

Now that it was clear that chlorophyll was the active agent in binding and eliminating some of the toxic pollutants, the next step was to find out how effectively chlorophyll-containing vegetables can lower toxic burden. When rats were fed a diet that was 10 percent vegetables, the higher the level of chlorophyll in the vegetables, the more toxins the rats eliminated. The vegetables that resulted in the smallest increase in dioxin excretion (60 percent to 300 percent increase) were Chinese cabbage, broccoli, green onion, Welsh onion, cabbage, and celery. Next highest (330 percent to 480 percent increase) were kale, Chinese chive, shungiku (edible chrysanthemum), green lettuce, and sweet peppers. The group that topped the charts with an increased dioxin excretion of 760 percent to 1,160 percent included komatsuna (Japanese mustard greens), mitsuba (Japanese wild parsley), spinach, and perilla (Japanese basil).

Obviously, spinach is the easiest chart topper to find at conventional grocery stores, but since it's also on the dirty dozen list, you'll need to find organic spinach or use some other form of chlorophyll. The same can be said for seaweeds. Though they're superstars when it comes to mobilizing toxins, they're also being found to be highly contaminated with heavy metals and aren't good candidates for adding to your diet. What would be a great addition is a combination of rice bran fiber (about 6 grams a day) and chlorophyll from a less-toxic source such as algae or greens such as organic kale (a brassica that also aids in liver function). But to get the most toxins out, it's important to use all of the body's elimination systems, including the kidneys.

Can't We Just Skip Fat Absorption in the First Place?

I've heard many people say, "Why can't they just invent a pill so we can eat whatever we want and not get fat?" Well, in a manner of speaking, that pill now exists.

As I briefly mentioned in chapter 3, your body breaks down the fats you eat with an enzyme called lipase, which is produced by the pancreas. The fats are digested with lipase in the small intestine, where they can then be absorbed so your body can make use of the nutrients and store away the rest. So right about now you might be thinking, wouldn't it be nice if there were some way not to absorb and store some of these fats? As it turns out, scientists are way ahead of you, having figured out that if you stop the pancreatic lipase from doing its job so efficiently, the fat you ingest becomes unabsorbable. And what the body can't absorb, it can't store. The fat has nowhere to go but out.

Alli, pharmaceutical giant GlaxoSmithKline's diet drug, works just this way. Orlistat, as it's officially known, is the most potent pancreatic lipase inhibitor available. It's so powerful that users are instructed to stick to a low-fat diet or beware the results. Too much fat moving too efficiently through the digestive system will result in the dreaded anal leakage. While the drug has inhibited fat absorption and led to weight loss in clinical trials, there has to be a better way.

Actually, there are plenty of natural alternatives to Alli. They work the same way—by curbing pancreatic lipase—but without the leakage and other side effects of the synthetic chemical version. Like Alli, they interfere with the body's ability to break down and absorb fat. The fat moves right on through the digestive system and out the other end without taking up residence anywhere along the way (such as, say, your hips). The inhibitors provide a "sink" for fat-soluble toxins to jump into and then carry them out with the fat. They don't inhibit as much of the pancreatic lipase as Alli does, though, so they work more slowly, and you don't have to worry about having an accident while you're out and about.

The natural lipase inhibitors include a number of common botanical agents such as horse chestnut (*Aesculus*), wild rose (*Rosa*), wild yam (*Dioscorea*), Asian ginseng (*Panax ginseng*), and tea (*Camellia sinensis*). These herbs all contain either saponins or polyphenols—both of which have weight-loss benefits—and other natural compounds. Saponins function as a plant's immune system, providing natural antibacterial and antifungal activity. And polyphenols are the active ingredients in tea that are responsible for all of the fantastic health benefits we've been hearing about, including cancer prevention.

All of these botanical agents have been shown to inhibit pancreatic lipase in animal models. The saponins from plants in the *Dioscorea* genus have dramatically reduced weight gain in rats fed a high–beef fat diet. When tested in mice alongside orlistat, saponins from Japanese ginseng and the orlistat both prevented the mice from gaining weight while on a high-fat diet and just about doubled their fecal-fat excretion. While they haven't been tested in a laboratory, horse chestnut seeds and wild rose leaves have the highest saponin content of any herb, so you could take smaller doses of these and get the same benefits.

Tea contains both polyphenols and saponins. The saponins in green tea seeds were able to inhibit lipase, prevent weight gain, and increase fecal-fat content in a 2001 study of animals on a high-fat diet. While saponins aren't found in a high amount in a cup of green tea, they are highly concentrated in the seeds and other parts of the plant and are available in many of the green tea supplements on the market. The good news for tea drinkers is that in addition to all of the other green tea benefits discussed in chapter 3, the polyphenol content aids in the excretion of fat-soluble toxins. In a study in which two groups of rats were exposed to PCBs and then put on a diet including either 4 grams of matcha green tea (the amount used to make two cups) or a placebo, those that consumed the matcha excreted over 4 times more PCBs than the placebo group did.

As for the polyphenols to be found in a cup of tea or three, a group of volunteers who drank polyphenol-rich oolong tea experienced over twice the amount of fecal-fat excretion as those who drank a placebo without polyphenols. The volunteers drank a cup containing 750 milliliters of tea three times a day, which is just a little more than what's found in three Starbucks venti-sized cups. And since oolong tea has less polyphenols than either green or white tea, you'd have to drink even less of those teas to get the same welcome benefits. Or you could drink the same amount and get even more benefits. By all means, drink up!

Clearing Toxins through Your Kidneys

We've talked about increasing the amount of toxins leaving the body through the bowels by blocking the recycling of toxins back into the bloodstream. The kidneys have a recycling system, too.

The biggest factor in how much of a toxic load your kidneys recycle is the pH (acid or alkaline levels) of your urine. The more acidic the urine, the more toxins are recycled. The more alkaline (or basic—the opposite of acidic) the urine, the less is recycled. Unfortunately, when the body becomes toxic, it also typically becomes more acidic. Eating foods we're reactive to also increases body acidity. In fact, the acidification of body tissues that this touches off is a major cause of many of the allergic symptoms we experience.

Cutting foods out of your diet that you're reactive to can go a long way toward alkalinizing your urine and increasing the amount of toxins leaving your body. Making other dietary changes that we've discussed, like piling more green vegetables onto your plate and cutting back on red meats and dairy, will also reduce your acidic level.

You can also alkalinize your urine by drinking sparkling water. For my evening "cocktail," I mix sparkling water with berry juice (blueberry and cranberry are my current favorites). All grocery stores carry sparkling water, and many have their own labels that cost less than the brand names. Some stores even offer discounts if you buy sparkling water by the case like my wife and I do.

There are also a number of herbal teas that help alkalinize the urine, such as stinging nettle (*Urtica dioica*). And a multiple vitamin-mineral combination whose minerals are in the citrate form (e.g., magnesium citrate and potassium citrate) will alkalinize your urine as well.

With your bowels moving regularly and your kidneys working well, the amount of toxins your body can eliminate will be exponentially increased. This alone will make you feel like a new person. But to make sure that your body is effectively handling not only the toxins but their by-products as well, it's important for you to make sure your liver is working at full capacity.

Optimize Your Liver Function

The liver is a critical link in the process of getting rid of the toxins that lead to weight gain. When any kind of chemical enters the bloodstream by way of our diet, the air, or our hormonal production, it's the liver's job to handle it. You might say your liver is your body's own personal bouncer.

During the first step of the process, conveniently called phase 1, a group of enzymes known as cytochromes begins breaking down toxins as they enter the liver. It's because of this initial breakdown that aspirin doesn't work longer than it does and a night of drinking doesn't keep us inebriated for more than a few hours. Whatever enters the bloodstream, be it caffeine, our own hormones, or paint fumes, will be metabolized into something else. Every tissue in the body except red blood cells and skeletal muscle has toxin-metabolizing enzymes that get this process rolling. The highest concentrations of these enzymes are in the small intestine and the lungs, where they go to work as soon as toxins enter the body, and in the liver, where they deal with whatever gets past those first lines of defense.

For phase 1 to be carried out properly — and to prepare your excess pounds for departure — certain nutrients have to be on board. These include the B vitamins, vitamin C, vitamin E, and the minerals magnesium and selenium. Over the years, I've found that I often have to administer very high levels of magnesium (up to 900 milligrams daily) and vitamin C (up to 12,000 milligrams daily) to my most toxic patients.

I also like to use multiple vitamins that have more thiamine, magnesium, and selenium than normal. These nutrients often lose the face-off with toxins, becoming deficient in our bodies while the toxins run rampant. Deficiencies of thiamine and selenium hinder phase 1 function and block our ability to recycle glutathione, one of the main molecules that escort chemicals from the body (it can also function as an antioxidant, after which it can be recycled and repurposed). I also look for a multiple vitamin that includes extracts of green tea, broccoli, *Taraxacum*, curcumin, and milk thistle, along with some alpha-lipoic acid and NAC. Diets high in protein and low in sugars and fats—similar to those Barry Sears recommends in *The Zone Diet*—also help phase 1 run smoothly. (See the resources at the back of this book for places to find such a multiple vitamin.)

As beneficial as the process is, the breaking down of toxins that occurs in phase 1 can't really be called detoxification because not everything is changed to a less toxic compound. I think that anyone who has ever experienced a hangover will agree that the metabolite of alcohol (aldehydes)—the substance produced when alcohol is metabolized—feels more toxic than the alcohol itself. Some compounds, such as the combustion byproduct BAP, are made into powerful cancer-causing compounds during phase 1. So, far from being out of the woods at this point, your body needs to keep hustling those toxins toward the exit.

In the next step, phase 2, another molecule is connected to the phase 1 metabolite to make it more water soluble and therefore easier to clear through the kidneys or the bowel. We can help the process along by providing nutrients for these toxins to bond with for easier excretion as well as nutrients that enhance the liver's ability to perform this wedding ceremony. Boosted levels of taurine (especially L-taurine), glutamine, and glycine are especially important for people exposed to solvents and those who are reactive to any solvent-based compound such as paints, glues, carpet, perfumes, soaps, and cleansers. People overloaded with these toxins are typically lacking in taurine, glutamine, and glycine, and because they bond with toxins, those nutrients are exactly what's needed.

As for boosting your glutathione, which clears combustion products, pesticides, and solvents, that's easily accomplished with the amino acid NAC. While many practitioners recommend oral capsules consisting of reduced glutathione molecules, the only published study on the capsules failed to show any increase in glutathione levels. NAC, on the other hand, has been documented to increase glutathione levels, as have whey protein supplements. And the higher the quality of whey, the better it is at making glutathione (and the more expensive it generally is). So making a daily smoothie with a high-quality whey protein goes a long way toward maintaining good glutathione levels.

As critical as glutathione levels are, though, they aren't sufficient in themselves to clear the body of toxins. Toxins and other chemicals that have undergone phase 1 breakdown in the liver also need properly functioning enzymes known as glutathione transferases (GSTs), which are what actually attach the glutathione to a toxic metabolite so it can then leave the body more easily. We have several types of GSTs in our bodies, and how efficiently we clear toxins often depends on how well they work. Fortunately, there are a number of botanical agents, including turmeric, green tea, and broccoli, that have beneficial effects on GST function (and in some cases glutathione levels as well).

Make More Good and Less Bad Estrogens

The liver is responsible for using metabolic enzymes to properly handle all of the chemical compounds we're exposed to. That includes hormones, medications, environmental toxins, and the natural beneficial chemicals in foods. But believe it or not, the liver's job doesn't end there—it also has to metabolize estrogens.

There's no doubt that the hormonal changes women experience when they go through menopause make it easier for them to gain weight and harder to lose it. But a healthy woman with a low toxic burden won't have nearly the same uphill battle as a woman like Victoria whose body was laden with toxins.

Foods and chemicals we ingest can influence the normal pathways through which estrogen is metabolized. Certain chlorinated pesticides and a combustion byproduct, for example, have been shown to boost production of the 16-OH estrogens (which can increase cancer risk) and slow production of the 2-OH estrogen (which can reduce cancer risk). Several things can be done naturally to cause estrogen metabolism to pump out more of the 2-OH and less of the 16-OH. Since combustion byproducts, chlorinated pesticides, and

PCBs have a negative effect on the ratio of good to bad estrogens, using the methods previously outlined in this book for avoiding further toxin exposure and reduction of your current load would be the best place to start.

Besides limiting exposure to persistent pollutants found in animal fat that increase cancer risk, diets low in fat can significantly curtail the production of 16-OH estrogens. Diets that have more protein and fewer carbohydrates than are found in the standard American diet also have been shown to improve estrogen ratios, as have soy products. In a study of women who drank soy milk every day, the levels of 2-OH estrogens increased by 27 percent, which greatly improved their good-to-bad ratio. When a soy-protein powder was given to another group of women, they experienced an increase in the good 2-OH production and a decrease in both 4-OH and 16-OH production. Apparently, it doesn't matter what kind of soy compound is used. And the dietary intake of broccoli and other brassicas has the same beneficial effect. So from a macro diet perspective, the best diet for balancing estrogen metabolism is a vegetarian one (low-fat, low-carb, high-protein, high-soy) with lots of broccoli. This isn't exactly hot news, but what is new is the ample evidence showing why this classic diet is so beneficial. If you're one of those people who are moaning, "But I hate broccoli"—chin up! I assure you there are ways you can eat it, drink it, and swallow it in pill form that you won't find objectionable.

In addition to the right basic diet choices, supplements can play a role in balancing estrogen metabolism. One is the herb rosemary. When mice were fed a diet that was 2 percent rosemary, their 2-OH production increased by a whopping 150 percent while their 16-OH levels dropped by 50 percent. Not bad for something that's a pleasure to eat. Flaxseed meal has also been known to work wonders. In a comparison with wheat bran, which showed no benefit, eating muffins with 10 grams of flaxseed caused a 34 percent increase in 2-OH levels. In another study, women ate either a muffin with 25 grams of soy flour or one with 25 grams of flaxseed every day for sixteen weeks; both groups saw improvements in their estrogen ratios, but the flaxseed group did significantly better, with a 103 percent increase in 2-OH levels. When postmenopausal women with primary breast cancer were given 25 grams of flaxseed a day, they also benefited.

After eating these muffins for a little over a month, their rates of cancer-cell death had accelerated and their cancer-cell production had slowed. So flaxseed meal appears to be beneficial in both preventing and treating breast cancers.

Making Sure Metabolized Estrogen Leaves Your Body

Once the phase 1 cytochromes have metabolized the estrogens, they need to go through phase 2 to be ready to leave the body. As with phase 1, there's more than one way out. The harmless 2-OH metabolites are quickly put through the methylation pathway—named for the methyl group that serves as ushers—and moved out of the body. The other metabolites—the ones with persistent estrogen activity—have two pathways available for the next step. In the sulfate pathway, a sulfur molecule attaches itself to the metabolites. Provided you have enough sulfur in your diet, commonly coming from eggs, onions, and garlic with the addition of some B vitamins and vitamin A, this pathway is very effective at ushering the sulfur-bound metabolites out of the body. But it's a different story for compounds that go through the other pathway.

In the liver, a variety of cancer-causing chemicals (including 16-OH estrogens), steroid hormones, and other toxins are bonded to glucuronic acid and then dumped into the intestines—that's the glucuronide pathway. Some of these compounds are recycled back into the blood, ideally to be removed by the kidneys or again cleared by the liver. But it's not always that easy. Enzymes called beta-glucuronidases, which are produced by certain intestinal bacteria, can break the bond between the chemical and its glucuronic acid transporter. This allows the chemical to be directed back into the bloodstream, where it has to be dealt with yet again (and can cause more problems). When this happens to the cancer-causing 16-OH estrogens, a higher risk of breast cancer is likely.

You're not defenseless, though. There's a natural compound called D-glucarate that can put a stop to this madness. It's the kryptonite that robs beta-glucuronidases of their power. If the body has high enough levels of this wonder compound known as D-glucarate, all of the metabolites that have bonded to glucuronic acid can be cleared via the stool or the urine. D-glucarates have been shown to protect against chemical-induced cancer in animals and to prevent lung and breast cancers and liver metastases from abdominal tumors.

A number of foods have high levels of D-glucarate, including the members of the Curcubitaceae family (squash, zucchini, pumpkin, melons), the Rosaceae family (apples, strawberries, cherries, plums, pears, blackberries, quince, loquats, currants) and the Leguminoceae family (beans, soy, lentils, peas, chickpeas). The more of these foods there are in your diet, the less active your beta-glucuronidase enzymes will be. The consumption of protein, fiber, and beta-carotene has also been shown to thwart the unwelcome enzymes. And the commercially available dietary supplement calcium D-glucarate has been used at levels of 1.5 to 9 grams a day in some studies to inhibit the enzymes.

The common herbs milk thistle and licorice also fight beta-glucuronidase. Milk thistle (*Silybum marianum*) is known as a formidable defender of the liver, and in some studies it's even proved its ability to protect against the toxic death cap mushroom and carbon tetrachloride—compounds that are usually surefire liver-killing chemicals. Besides these impressive abilities, milk thistle can curtail the activity of intestinal beta-glucuronidases by over 50 percent. And glycyrrhizin, a main component of licorice, also has the capacity to shut these enzymes down, which is undoubtedly why it's able to prevent liver cancer after exposure to carbon tetrachloride. The probiotics *Lactobacillus acidophilus* and *Bifidobacterium* are other powerful foes of beta-glucuronidase.

So when it comes to preventing the recycling of cancer-causing chemicals, including estrogens, you can get great benefit from a diet high in fruits and vegetables; and even greater benefit by adding licorice, milk thistle, and good probiotics to the menu.

Besides the supplements I've already mentioned (sources for which can be found in the resource section of this book), a host of others can support your body in its quest to become a lean, green, well-oiled machine. I'll focus on them in the next chapter.

CHAPTER 5

Supplements: Your Secret Weapons

Every day at noon I saw Erminia leaning heavily on the counter at the deli where she worked. She wasn't more than 5 feet 5 inches tall, but she must have tipped the scales at 280 pounds, maybe even 300. So it wasn't surprising that she didn't have the energy to stand up straight.

The deli had the best healthy lunch in the area, so I was a regular customer and over time Erminia and I got to know each other a little. I noticed when she started to lose weight—it was obvious—and she was ecstatic that the new diet she was on was working. She'd dropped a few sizes and told me her blood pressure had gone down a little, too. She felt great all around. Until she didn't. Soon Erminia began to feel ill—exhausted, achy, headachy. And she certainly didn't feel up to exercising.

One day when I went into the shop, Erminia told me she'd just had her blood pressure checked and it was sky-high. I suggested she stop by my clinic and let me see whether I could help with the problem. Fortunately, she did.

Erminia was only forty-nine, but when I tested her not only was her blood pressure high, but so were her cholesterol and blood sugar levels.

After we talked for a while and I told her she could be feeling much better very soon, she committed to making a change. "Everything you said about how I've been feeling is true, Dr. Crinnion," she said. "Enough's enough. Tell me what I need to do."

I told her to begin by cutting out unhealthy carbs and starting to get regular aerobic exercise. I asked her to begin walking for twenty minutes a day and to find out whether there was a pool nearby that she could walk and exercise in. On her own, she also decided to join a local gym where she could feel comfortable working out with other women who were about her age and size.

I recognized the negative cycle Erminia had been sucked into every time she'd gone on a diet. As she'd begin to lose weight, the toxins stored in her fat tissues would be released into her body. She wasn't sick exactly—she was poisoned. Her body needed to clear out the toxins so they wouldn't be circulating and making her feel so lousy.

I began Erminia on the program that would escort fat-soluble toxins out of the body and started her on the nutrients to be discussed in this chapter. Within six weeks of being on the program, she felt fine, started exercising again, and was eating right. This time the pounds fell off more quickly and easily than before—60 pounds over the next ten months—with no return of her symptoms. Her blood sugar dropped, too, along with her blood pressure and cholesterol level. And her energy level was through the roof. As of this writing, Erminia was still on the program and still losing weight at the healthy rate of about 1 or 2 pounds a week.

There are plenty of natural ways to supplement a diet to usher fat-soluble compounds out of the body like Erminia did. In the previous chapters, we discussed some of the biggies: fibers, chlorophyll, saponins, and polyphenols. Once you've opened the exit routes with those compounds, you can begin to safely increase the amount of the toxins that are dumped from their storage space in your fat. This can be accomplished with chlorophyll products, rice bran fiber, green tea, and colonic irrigations as you learned in chapter 4 (these methods are also listed in the resource section of this book). But there are also vitamins, herbs, oils, and spices that will protect your body while the toxins make their way out, and there are nutrients you can take to help your liver do its very important detox work. I'll introduce you to these natural wonders — and a "miracle" vegetable — in this chapter, and in week four of the clean, green, and lean plan I'll provide you with a prescriptive list and explain how much to take.

As with all aspects of life, the closer we align our behavior with our goals, the sooner we achieve those goals. If your goal is to safely and effectively lose weight and reduce your total toxic burden, you're going to need different supplements from what you'd need if your goal were simply to find a multivitamin that's appropriate for your age.

If you just wanted to know the most important vitamins to take to ensure general good health, you could check any number of books already on the market. But this program goes beyond that. The supplements I recommend include all of the basic nutrients you need to be healthy, of course, but the main goals are to protect your body against toxins and have them escorted right out of your body along with fats.

Taking the recommended clean, green, and lean supplements will ensure that you get adequate nutrients that tend to be deficient in people whose bodies are burdened with toxins and fat. These supplements are your secret weapons in the battle of the bulge. They protect your cells and tissues from toxin damage and properly clear toxins from your bloodstream.

Most people don't want to take a bunch of supplements, and I don't blame them. But with the burden of toxicity that most of us have to deal with, on average we need to take about two dozen. The number of capsules I take every day with my breakfast is twenty-three. I do this because of all I know about the environment and my body, and judging by my recent checkups, they're working great. All of the visits have ended with the physicians telling me I have the health of a man half my age. That's pretty good considering that I come from a family that's rampant with heart disease (my father had his first heart attack at age forty-eight). While I don't particularly enjoy swallowing a lot of capsules, I just look at them as the "price of admission" for a physically healthy life in a very toxic world. And it's a lot easier to swallow a few handfuls of pills than to end up suffering a coronary and then having to go through surgery and rehab. And it's a lot cheaper than the hospital bill would be for all that care.

The supplement program I recommend is built around a top-quality multivitamin with minerals and high levels of the vitamins C, A, and E, which are crucial antioxidants. The program also includes levels of some nutrients that are higher than what's found in many multivitamins, as well as some more unusual ingredients. In week four, you'll learn what to look for on your multivitamin label and learn about some other vitamins and minerals you should take.

Toxin-Fighting Multivitamins
- Vitamin B1
- Vitamin B2
- Vitamin B6
- Magnesium
- Alpha-lipoic acid
- N-acetyl-L-cysteine (NAC)
- Selenium

In addition to those critical vitamins and minerals, there are other supplements that support your body's detox and weight-loss process. I call these the most valuable players (MVPs).

Meet Your MVPs

It would be wonderful if we could get all of the nutrients that we need from our diet, but in all my years of practice I have met only one person who got even the recommended daily allowance (RDA) of basic nutrients. The RDA is based on the amount of each nutrient that we need to keep us from becoming nutritionally deficient—a far cry from what we need for optimal health. My sole patient who reached the RDA for her nutrients, based on a computerized diet analysis, spent every day growing and making her own foods. Every day, all day! But even she was short of the level of nutrients needed for optimal health.

The RDA doesn't take into account the extra need for certain nutrients that the toxic environment causes. So here is what each of us really needs more of.

Vitamin C

Also known as ascorbic acid, vitamin C is a water-soluble vitamin that's exceptionally easy to absorb and can be taken in quite high doses. It has a venerable history and was made famous in the 1980s when Dr. Linus Pauling (the only person to receive two Nobel prizes in a lifetime) pioneered its use for treating terminal cancer patients and preventing the common cold. By using doses of 20 grams or more a day (20,000 milligrams), he was able to keep terminal cancer patients alive for much longer than others with the same cancers who didn't dose up on vitamin C. Those who have followed in Pauling's footsteps have also shown how vitamin C can help prevent the occurrence of cardiovascular disease (heart attacks). Dr. John Ely, a brilliant researcher at the University of Washington, told me years ago: "Ten grams of vitamin C on the first day of a cold always works. After that it never works." I've found his words to be true, as have many of my patients.

Vitamin C is vital for the proper functioning of our white blood cells, which fight off the invading bacteria and viruses that lead to colds and flu. Eating sugar and smoking cigarettes robs our bodies of this invaluable nutrient. So does breathing in toxic air in cities. It's been estimated that one cigarette uses up as much as 200 milligrams of vitamin C. This might not sound like much, but the RDA for vitamin C is only 60 milligrams—the amount needed to keep us from developing scurvy!

Vitamin C is also necessary for the functioning of the phase 1 enzymes in the liver, enhancing the clearance of toxins from the bloodstream; a deficiency of vitamin C leads to diminished clearance from the blood and greater toxic effects. Besides aiding in clearance, vitamin C helps increase the excretion of these compounds from the body. And along with vitamin E, vitamin C also protects us from the lung damage that ozone causes. So if you live in a city, especially if you're a runner or a cyclist, you need to be taking vitamin C daily. I tell people that if they live in a city, they should take at least 3,000 milligrams of vitamin C a day. And if they're smokers or are in traffic a lot, they should double that amount.

Vitamin C is also important for excretion and the production of bile acids, which are toxins' actual means of transport out of the liver. In a study of guinea pigs (the other mammals besides humans that don't manufacture their own vitamin C), short-term vitamin C deficiency reduced the levels of vitamin C in the liver by 25 percent and led to a 50 percent reduction in both the amount produced and the effectiveness of the bile that was present.

In a word, vitamin C is indispensable. I've been taking 4,000 milligrams a day for the past twenty years.

Whey Protein Powder

Another MVP is whey protein powder. In chapter 4, I discussed how protein helps improve the clearance of toxins and medications from the bloodstream and inhibits some of the pancreatic lipase in the small intestine, which breaks fat down for absorption. Well, whey protein provides a great way to get some protein into your body and has the distinction of being the only one of the protein powders that raises levels of glutathione, which escort toxins from the body. This makes whey protein a fantastic addition to any program.

Whey is one of the proteins in dairy that's removed when milk is made into cheese. Many people are reactive to dairy, but not all of them are reactive to whey. If you have an adverse reaction to both milk and cheese, you're probably not reactive to whey, since whey isn't in cheese. But if you react to milk and not to cheese, you may be reactive to whey. If you're not sure, you can go to a licensed naturopathic physician to do a blood test for food allergies.

There's a great deal of difference in quality among the various whey proteins out there. You can gauge their quality just by checking the price differences. As with all supplements—and clothes and cars and everything else—you get what you pay for. If you buy supplements based on price alone and automatically go for the least expensive, you'll typically get the worst-absorbed and least bioavailable nutrients. In other words, you're spending hard-earned money on ingredients that your body isn't going to absorb and that will just end up in the toilet without having benefited you at all. When looked at in that light, the lower-priced supplements are actually the most expensive in terms of the return on your investment. It's no different with whey powder. While it's composed entirely of whey, the way it's processed makes a huge difference in how well it mixes and its ability to make glutathione in your body. The highest-quality products are all sold through consumer-direct companies and not through health food stores. These products are all processed under high pressure at low temperatures so that the disulfide bonds remain intact. It's these intact bonds that are used to make glutathione in the body. The lower-cost whey powders provide protein but don't have these intact bonds that are critical in our battle against our toxic burden. Repeated studies have shown that about 45 grams of high-quality whey a day is needed to really boost glutathione levels.

Probiotics

While you're shopping for whey, why not stop by the refrigerated section and pick up some healthy bacteria? I bet no one's ever said that to you before. But believe it or not, you really can—and should—buy bacteria.

Your bowels are inhabited by millions of healthy bacteria that help you stay healthy. When you take antibiotics, these healthy bacteria can be killed in large numbers. They can be replaced by aggressive pathogenic (illness-causing) bacteria that you'd really rather not have inside you. When you're stressed, the immune system "police officers" that take care of your intestines are present in far fewer numbers than normal, and the bad bacteria or yeasts can overgrow. These pathogenic invaders can cause a lot of havoc for your intestines and your body as a whole. Pick up any book on the effects of *Candida albicans* and you can read all about the far-reaching effects of this little organism.

Since your bowels are under toxin attack along with the rest of your body, it's wise to take special care of them. The two most commonly used healthy bacteria strains—or probiotics—are *Lactobacillus acidophilus* and *Bifidobacteria bifidus*.

Bifidobacteria bifidus is the predominant healthy bacteria in infants and children. It's also very effective at helping clear the class of chemicals known as aldehydes from the blood (*Lactobacillus* GG strain is also effective for this). The result of the breakdown of alcohol, aldehydes are the cause of hangovers. They're also the toxin that *Candida albicans* produces and releases into the body, and they're in formaldehyde as well. So if you've had a close encounter with any of these issues, you'd benefit from taking *B. bifidus*.

But these bacterial supplements appear to have even more powerful things going for them. In a study of more than nine hundred people in the United States with severe multiple chemical sensitivity, the researchers rated the effectiveness of various supplements, treatments, and environments. Not surprisingly, what benefited 95 percent of the participants the most was living in chemically safe homes (see chapter 6). But the supplement that had the highest helpful rating was probiotics. The use of probiotics appears to have real power to help lower levels of circulating toxins.

The notion that healthy bacteria help reduce the level of toxins in the body is borne out by a study conducted in an area of China where liver cancer is prevalent because of the presence of the mold *Aspergillus* in the food supply. The study showed that those who used *Lactobacillus* probiotic supplements were at lower risk for liver cancer. The researchers said the probiotics blocked the intestines from absorbing the cancer-causing mold toxins.

Probiotics are heavy hitters indeed. When they work alongside vitamin C, whey protein, and the other MVP supplements such as rice bran fiber and chlorophyll (covered in chapter 4) you have a dream team going to bat for you.

Give a Warm Welcome to the Top Fat Fighters

If you need help mobilizing fat so that your weight drops and you move more toxins from storage into the blood and intestines for removal, these extra nutrients can be exceedingly helpful.

Green Tea

When I first told Erminia about drinking green tea, she scrunched up her face and told me she hated tea—no matter what color it was. But when I told her she could lose weight by relaxing with a warm fruity or spicy beverage, feet up on the sofa, I had her attention. Really, people, how hard is it to drink a cup of tea? Find a few flavors of green tea you like and let them work their magic while you take a break.

In addition to green tea's ability to clear nasty toxins from the body, it can aid weight loss, which we know releases stored toxins into the bloodstream so that they can then be eliminated from the body. (White tea is great, too, by the way, though not as readily available.) To find out how effective is it as a weight-loss product, a group of forty-six women were put on a low-calorie diet and given either green tea extract (GTE) or a placebo. The first phase of the study lasted for thirty-two days, during which those taking the GTE lost 21 percent of their prestudy weight (someone starting at a weight of 250 pounds would have ended up at 198). As they continued for fifty-five more days, they didn't just maintain the weight loss—they lost 7 percent more. In another study, seventy-six overweight men and women used GTE with caffeine (for a total of 270 milligrams of the main catechin compound in green tea and 150 milligrams of caffeine) or a placebo every day. Those who took the extract (which was their only source of caffeine) lost weight, but they lost less than those who had a higher daily dose of caffeine. Caffeine does increase our metabolic rate, the rate at which we burn calories, and this is probably why having the caffeine helped. So if you want the weight-loss effect of green tea, don't drink decaffeinated teas.

Capsaicin: The Hottest Fat Fighter

If you don't like to eat hot peppers, don't worry, the essential fat-fighting ingredient and the source of the hot peppers' heat—capsaicin—is available as a supplement. In a capsaicin research study, participants took a supplement of 0.4 milligram of capsaicin and 625 milligrams of GTE (containing 125 milligrams of catechins and 50 milligrams of caffeine). After just two weeks, they showed a significant decrease in their body-fat percentage (an average of a pound) and an increase in their resting rate of thermogenesis, an increase that will continue to promote slow weight loss for as long as the extract is taken. This isn't very much capsaicin, so if you don't mind eating spicy foods, you should be able to get this amount easily by adding hot peppers to your meal. Those who can't handle the heat can check the resource section of this book or just look for a capsule version at the health food store.

The benefit of adding capsaicin to your diet apparently comes from its ability to enhance fat breakdown. When a group of ninety-one overweight people ate a low-calorie diet for four weeks and were then given either a capsule of capsaicin or a placebo, the group taking the capsaicin experienced more fat breakdown than the placebo group. Though capsaicin alone wasn't sufficient to prevent the return of weight after the monthlong diet, when taken with a thermogenic product such as caffeine, it offers a nice benefit.

Conjugated Linoleic Acid

The third fat fighter I recommend is conjugated linoleic acid (CLA). CLA is a mixture of different forms of linoleic acid, which is an essential omega-6 oil, and it's been shown to safely reduce fat levels and increase lean body mass. In six-, twelve- and twenty-four-month studies conducted in Norway, participants could eat whatever they wanted in whatever quantities they chose, and no lifestyle changes were required. In the six-month study, 118 people took either 3 or 4 grams of CLA a day or a placebo, and all of those who took CLA experienced significant weight loss. While the greatest reduction occurred in the legs, women who took CLA also enjoyed a big improvement in their waist-to-hip ratios. In the twelve-month study, two groups took 4.5 grams of CLA (in two different forms), while a third group took a placebo (4.5 grams of olive oil). The results: the CLA groups lost 7 to 9 percent more of their body-fat mass than the placebo group did. These losses were accomplished without the aid of other dietary measures or exercise. After that study, 125 of the 180 men and women who'd participated in it signed up for another twelve months. During this second year, they used only 3.4 grams of CLA a day, with the placebo again being olive oil. The final results: the CLA group maintained the weight loss that had been achieved in the first year. No adverse effects were noted among any of the groups taking the CLA.

All of these studies, by the way, were randomized, double-blind studies, the kind that we researchers and clinicians love to see. In this case, such safeguards mean that it wasn't just some random coincidence—it was without a doubt the CLA that caused the weight loss.

Liver Boosters: Herbs and Spices

All of these herbs and spices will enhance the clearance of toxins from your bloodstream and protect your liver from chemical damage. In the four-week plan, you'll be incorporating one or more of these into your daily diet. These liver boosters are all available in supplement form.

Rooibos

The African herb *Aspalanthus linearis*, known commonly as rooibos—or red bush—has been shown to increase the level of glutathione in the liver and enhance the functioning of liver enzymes. These properties make rooibos (pronounced ROY-bosch) a superb botanical agent in the body's fight against toxicity, but its beneficial effects on the liver go beyond improving its metabolism—it also protects and regenerates the liver.

In a study where rats were given the chemical carbon tetrachloride (CCL4)—the best-known liver-killing compound next to the death cap mushroom (*Amanita phalloides*)—the condition of their livers improved dramatically when they were also given rooibos. The herb actually brought about a reversal of the chemical-induced fatty liver that was present. In chapter 2, I reviewed a study showing that repeated weight loss and gain resulted in the development of fatty liver, a condition in which chlorinated toxins are concentrated in the liver and which is linked to increased rates of liver disease and diabetes. Rooibos would be well worthwhile even if reversing fatty liver were its only amazing feat, but the benefits revealed in the CCL4 study also included a reversal of the state of cirrhosis and diminished liver damage.

Rosemary

Another of nature's soldiers in the war on toxins is rosemary (*Rosmarinus officinalis*), a wonderfully fragrant shrub that's as sublime in food as it is powerful in the body. Like rooibos, rosemary was tested on rats exposed to CCL4, and it proved to be just as effective. Rosemary was able to partially prevent the inflammation and cell death (necrosis) caused by CCL4. The herb also boosted the activity of enzymes in both the liver and the blood, primarily the ones that handle combustion by-products and alcohol.

For women, rosemary has other benefits as well. As was discussed in chapter 4, estrogens can be metabolized into different end products: the beneficial 2-OH estrogen metabolites and the 4-OH and 16-OH compounds, which are associated with increased breast-cancer risk. So it's best for a woman to make more 2-OH metabolites of her estrogens than the 4- or 16-OH, and taking a rosemary extract is one of the natural steps that leads in this direction. Rosemary has been shown to increase 2-OH production by 150 percent while cutting back on the bad 16-OH estrogen metabolites by 50 percent.

Rosemary extracts can also head off damage to various tissues in the body. It can prevent lung cells from undergoing the genetic changes that lead to cancer after exposure to the main carcinogen in cigarette smoke and car emissions (BAP). It's also been shown to prevent damage from the very potent toxin aflatoxin B1, which enters the body as a result of eating contaminated peanut butter and leads directly to liver cancer. (Peanut butter can become contaminated when peanut shells bearing the mold *Aspergillus* are ground up with the peanuts.)

So besides protecting against lung cancer, rosemary can help fend off liver cancer. To top it off, rosemary also has a long history of helping the brain—specifically with improved memory—probably due to its antioxidant properties. Recently, it's been shown to protect brain cells against the toxic effects of rotenone (a natural pesticide, one that comes from nature, not from a chemical plant, and one that organic gardeners use), which is one of the chemical compounds known to cause Parkinson's disease. Rosemary hasn't been tested against other toxic environmental chemicals known to cause the neurologic damage that leads to parkinsonism, but since the damage appears to be the same, it's likely that this superherb can lend a hand there, too.

Dandelion

Another powerful herb is considered nothing more than a pesky weed by homeowners and golf course groundskeepers across the country. But such prejudices aside, dandelion (*Taraxacum officinale*) has a lot going for it, including the B vitamin choline, which helps in phase 1 liver function. It's also helpful for other liver problems, such as jaundice, cirrhosis, and high cholesterol. In addition to helping it clear toxins from the bloodstream, dandelion helps the liver produce and dump bile. In one study, rats that drank a mix of water and 2 percent *Taraxacum* tea experienced a whopping 244 percent increase in the functioning of one of the phase 2 enzymes.

Milk Thistle

Milk thistle's active component, silymarin, uses three mechanisms to protect the liver:

- It binds to the outer membrane of liver cells to protect them from chemical damage.
- It contributes powerful antioxidant activity that adds to cellular protection and ensures quenching of harmful free radicals.
- It helps in the regeneration of damaged liver cells. Yes, it actually can get damaged liver cells to heal!

By binding to the outer membranes of liver cells, silymarin acts as a shield, protecting them from damaging chemicals and toxins. This was dramatically illustrated in studies examining silymarin's defenses against the death cap mushroom, whose toxins cause swift and severe damage to the liver. Because it binds to the sites on the liver cells where these toxins would normally latch on, silymarin headed off all damage.

When silymarin was administered before death cap poisoning, it was 100 percent effective in preventing toxicity. Even when given ten minutes after the toxin, it completely counteracted the toxic effects. If given within twenty-four hours, silymarin would still prevent death and greatly reduce the amount of liver damage. It's so powerful that an injectable form of silibin—the major component of silymarin—has become a mainstay in German emergency rooms for treatment of such poisoning.

Silymarin works as a powerful antioxidant in the liver cells as well as in the stomach and intestines. This is primarily due to its ability to both increase the amount of glutathione in the liver and make sure it's used as efficiently as possible. Research indicates that silymarin's antioxidant properties are ten times more powerful than vitamin E's—which is saying something. Silymarin also helps the liver by stabilizing cell membranes, making them more resistant to damage, and regenerating liver cells that have been damaged.

Among the conditions silymarin has been useful in treating are liver damage caused by drug and alcohol abuse, acute and chronic hepatitis, and cirrhosis. Clinical use has indicated that it may help prevent gallstones as well and is useful in the treatment of skin conditions like psoriasis and acne that can be cleared up only if the liver is functioning healthily. Studies have also shown that silymarin can inhibit the production of inflammatory chemicals in the body and reverse the symptoms of alcoholism, including weakness, loss of appetite, and nausea.

Turmeric (*Curcuma longa*)

Turmeric is a major component of curry powder and is used in some prepared mustards. It's also used in both Chinese and ayurvedic medicine as an anti-inflammatory herb and in the treatment of many conditions. Turmeric has repeatedly demonstrated its ability to protect the liver from a number of powerful liver toxins, including CCL4, aflatoxin, and alcohol. It can also boost phase 2 enzymes and glutathione.

Antioxidants: Your Body's Cellular-Service Providers

All environmental chemicals cause oxidative damage when they enter our bodies and transform into free radicals that rob our cells and tissues of precious electrons. This oxidative damage is what leads to chronic diseases like heart disease and to the changes in our bodies that we attribute to aging. Since these compounds target our brains, our blood vessels, the mitochondria in each cell, and all of our organs, I strongly recommend that you begin taking lots of protective antioxidants. Walking around in today's world without taking antioxidants is like walking into a burning building without an oxygen mask.

The most damaging event for our mitochondria is an overload of oxidative compounds—the mitochondria have no means of protecting themselves from this assault. So any increase in antioxidant levels will ultimately help our mitochondria, but some antioxidants help protect mitochondria more than others.

Vitamin E

Vitamin E is a well-known stabilizer of cell membranes as well as a potent antioxidant. This fat-soluble vitamin has been shown to prevent respiratory damage from ozone and lessen the toxic effects of other chemicals on the body.

For years, vitamin E has been used to reduce the risk of heart disease. While some articles have questioned its value to heart health, a study of almost thirty thousand Finnish men showed that those with the highest vitamin E levels had the lowest death rates. And women who took vitamin E had a much lower risk for experiencing sudden death from cardiovascular disease or blood clots.

Vitamin E has also been shown to prevent chemicals from damaging the mitochondria and to restore mitochondrial function. The chemicals it was tested against in those studies are among those that lead to Parkinson's disease. Other studies have shown that people with another chronic brain disease, Alzheimer's, have lower levels of vitamin E in their brains than people without the disease.

Ginkgo Biloba

This herb has a long history of helping to improve brain function, including memory. It does a number of things that boost the functioning of the brain cells, including serving as a potent antioxidant, enhancing blood flow to the brain, and enhancing brain cells' ability to get glucose from the blood. (Anyone who has experienced the severe brain fog that comes with low blood sugar can tell you how important sugar is to brain cells.) It's also a powerful antioxidant for the mitochondria, protecting them from damage.

Berry Extracts

Berry extracts are another potential supplement to your diet with antioxidant properties that are well worth harnessing and putting to work for you. Besides being delicious—ask Erminia—blackberry is one of the few compounds that have been shown to greatly enhance antioxidant activity and actually reverse mitochondrial damage. All of the berries with similar dark blue coloring have powerful antioxidant activity, but blackberries appear to be the most active. If you're serious about optimizing your mitochondrial functioning—and I hope I've made clear how critical it is to heal yourself by starting with your cells' building blocks—you'll add blackberry to your supplement regimen.

Elderberry

Elderberry offers a different twist on antioxidants' invaluable benefits. Anthocyanins, the antioxidants in elderberry, can be incorporated *into* the cells that line the blood vessels (endothelial cells). This protects the cells from oxidative damage, including damage from hydrogen peroxide and the oxidizing of excess iron in the body that is associated with increased risk of heart disease and some infective processes. In the case of the latter, this protection could allow you to take an iron-containing supplement without increasing your risk of heart disease, which has been linked to oxidizing iron. Elderberry extracts can also curb the oxidation of LDL cholesterol, the bad cholesterol that leads to heart disease. This is a huge benefit in the prevention of heart disease and one of its precursors, atherosclerosis, since oxidation of LDL is thought to be the main cause of these problems.

Elderberry is a tall treelike shrub native to Europe, Asia, and North Africa that, fortunately, has taken root in the United States and can be found growing wild here. Besides being an antioxidant, it's a potent supporter of the immune system—one of the other body systems targeted for damage by environmental toxins. Elderberry extracts can significantly enhance white blood cells' response to an invading organism. It pulls this off by stepping up the production of chemical messengers called cytokines that literally turn on the body's immune response. When it comes to viral fighting, elderberry is a legendary scrapper. Extracts have shown the ability to fight colds and keep the herpes simplex type 1 virus from multiplying. In the laboratory, it has also proved capable of lessening the infectivity of both HIV and the H1N1 swine flu virus. And in studies assessing elderberry extract's effect on people with the flu, those who took elderberry extract recovered their health in less than half the time that the placebo group did.

Wolfberry

Wolfberry (*Lycium barbarum*) is a powerful antioxidant that prevents the development of atherosclerosis and heart disease. Several articles have shown that wolfberry is also an excellent source of the antioxidant zeaxanthin, which is believed to combat eye disorders.

In one study, wolfberry extracts led to a reduction in the levels of blood sugar, triglycerides, and cholesterol in animals whose levels had been elevated. The improved blood sugar balance was probably due to wolfberry's beneficial effects on the mitochondria. Meanwhile, the levels of good cholesterol, HDL, increased. With heart disease and diabetes at epidemic proportions, these are benefits that most people need. In that sense, it shouldn't be regarded as a supplement but as a staple of our diets. It is for Erminia. After seeing her blood sugar and cholesterol levels plummet after taking wolfberry, she was converted for life.

Since we know that mitochondrial damage leads to fatigue, it shouldn't come as a shock to find that wolfberry has also shown promise on that front. As an energy booster, it just might turn out to be something of a miracle drug for people who regularly engage in strenuous work. In one study, the extract was shown to aid in the body's ability to handle intensified exercise and resist fatigue. It also enhanced short-term energy storage—a bonus for athletes—and helped clear metabolic-breakdown products from the blood after exercise.

As with the other antioxidants in this section, wolfberry is also beneficial to the immune system. In the laboratory, wolfberry extract has been shown to enhance the responsiveness of the immune system in general and specifically the white blood cells responsible for fighting viruses. It can also support macrophages—the white blood cells' sentinels—in their mission to alert the rest of the immune system that an invader is in their midst. This is a crucial step in starting the immune response. If the macrophages aren't up to the job, the result is an unresponsive immune system, which leads to chronic viral and fungal infections. Mercury, which is in all of us, has been shown to chip away at the macrophages' powers, and fortunately we have wolfberrry to help reverse that.

Wolfberry is also on the front line in the fight against toxic chemicals. It's been shown to head off liver damage from CCL4 and prevent depletion of glutathione levels in the liver. It has also proved comparable to milk thistle in its liver-protection abilities. Finally, it can reverse the suppression of bone marrow by toxic chemicals and bring about an increase in circulating red blood cells, white blood cells, and platelets.

My wife and I take a liquid extract every day that contains wolfberry as well as green tea, broccoli, elderberry, blackberry, and mangosteen. We love it and it provides us with great mitochondrial support and protection in addition to helping us reduce our toxic load. The resource section lists the company we get it from.

L-carnitine and Coenzyme Q10

Two more power hitters in the antioxidant lineup are L-carnitine and coenzyme Q10 (CoQ10). L-carnitine is an amino acid that ushers fats through the cells to the mitochondria where they can be used for fuel. The food with the highest concentration of L-carnitine is avocado, which happens to be on the clean dozen list. The mitochondria also need CoQ10 for proper functioning. This wonderful nutrient has proved its worth in cases of high blood pressure, mitral valve prolapse, and congestive heart failure (a definite mitochondrial malfunction). It's also the only nutrient known to slow the progression of Parkinson's disease. Because Parkinson's results from mitochondrial dysfunction, some smart researchers put CoQ10 on the case to see what would happen. They gave people in the early stages of parkinsonism one of three different daily levels of CoQ10—300 milligrams, 600 milligrams, or 1,200 milligrams—for sixteen months. They found that the disease's progress was slowed the most for those taking the highest dose.

Broccoli: In a Class of Its Own

From what I have learned and witnessed in my patients, broccoli is no less than a superpower when it comes to being clean, green, and lean.

Broccoli is a variety of *Brassica oleracea*. Other varieties include cauliflower, brussels sprouts, kohlrabi, kale, and cabbage. Among their many nutrients are two major classes of health-promoting chemical compounds: sulforaphanes and indole-3-carbinols. The indole-3-carbinols help the body to metabolize estrogens in a healthy way, increasing the production of safe 2-OH estrogen metabolites and suppressing potentially dangerous 16-OH metabolites. But for now, let's consider the impressive benefits of the sulforaphanes.

Thanks to sulforaphanes, eating broccoli can dramatically reduce the risk of colorectal cancer (by 82 percent), prostate cancer (by 42 percent), breast cancer (by 40 percent), and lung cancer (by 39 percent). These being some of the most common cancers, it would be wise for us all to eat our broccoli and its *Brassica* relatives on a daily basis. You're not sold? How about this: broccoli can also increase the clearance of toxins from the body (which may be a major factor in its cancer-fighting powers). You still don't want to eat it every day? Think about this: if you eat broccoli every other day, it's protecting you only half as much as it could. Eat broccoli just once a week, and it's protecting you only a seventh as much. In the scheme of things, eating broccoli every day seems like a small price to pay. This is especially true since we're taking in toxins every day. For those of you still holding out, see the resources for information on finding broccoli extracts, which, being tasteless, should do the trick. My wife and I love to eat it, and we get it in our daily "Liquid Life" extract that's also in the resource section.

Multiple research articles have shown that broccoli boosts one of the phase 1 enzymes that help clear our blood of caffeine and some of the combustion products we breathe. It also lends a hand to phase 2 enzymes, even for those who have one of the polymorphisms that lead to impaired liver function. People who have one of those genetic differences we discussed earlier have a higher rate of many diseases, including cancers, but when they eat broccoli regularly, certain enzymes crank up and pick up the slack for those that don't work so well.

Now that you understand how being clean and green naturally leads to being lean, you're ready to embark on the four-week plan.

CHAPTER 6

Your Home on a Diet

When I first met my patient Sal, I couldn't believe he'd come to see me about weight loss. He was thirty-eight years old and about 6 feet tall, and he weighed 210 pounds. For his height and body type, he was at most 15 pounds overweight, but he said he'd been trying to lose those 15 pounds for the past four years with no success. He'd tried liquid diet shakes, frozen low-fat dinners, and giving up carbs, but he couldn't get rid of the fat that had accumulated around his midsection. In talking with Sal, I learned that he'd been getting hives on his hands and feet at night and had been taking antihistamines on a somewhat regular basis. I also learned that he'd moved into a new house a few years earlier. As the information added up, it all pointed to one thing: a toxic environment. Sal's house was storing toxins, and the little bit of fat he was carrying was stubbornly holding on to those toxins.

When I told Sal that it was his house—not him—that we had to put on a diet, he burst out laughing. The idea that the furniture, carpeting, and a variety of common household items such as bug spray were keeping him from losing weight sounded like one of the most ridiculous things he'd ever heard. But when I explained to him that the toxins were not only making it hard for him to lose weight but were also slowing down his metabolism, I had his attention.

For Sal to lose weight and eliminate his allergic reactions, he had to scale back the amount of environmental toxins he was exposed to, especially the ones in his home. He worked out of a home office, so that's where he spent most of his time, and those were the environmental toxins he had the most control over.

When I give a talk at a seminar or appear on a TV show, the audience members are always aghast when they hear about the poisons that are right under their noses in their own homes. They're shocked to learn that products they use to kill germs and get rid of dirt are much more lethal to them than the germs and dirt themselves. What happened that has made people think we have to wage toxic warfare on common household dust and dirt? My grandmother could clean just about anything with water, vinegar, or baking soda. Today, those are among my own preferred cleaning products. And they don't take much longer to use. When I'm in the shower, I use a squeegee to clean the walls. It takes only a minute and prevents soap scum buildup that would require either a lot of elbow grease or the use of a nasty solvent. It's well worth the effort, and it keeps the glass looking good, too.

"Americans breathe in at least as much nasty stuff as they eat, if not more," I told Sal. "The toxins get into the cells all the same—they don't care which door they go in through. So you need to protect yourself from them just as vigilantly."

At this, Sal looked a little doubtful again. He couldn't believe companies are allowed to sell products that are so lethal. "Be straight with me," he said. "I mean, how evil can a cup of fabric softener be?"

I could understand his skepticism. I'd heard it countless times from other patients. They're dumbfounded when they learn that slapping a warning label on a toxic product is sometimes all companies have to do. When I told Sal this, he said, "Well, I knew I wasn't supposed to drink the stuff, but I didn't know that smelling it could hurt me." I explained that detoxing the home along with the diet is essential if a person wants to lose weight and get rid of chemical sensitivity.

Once Sal understood the importance of kicking these products out of his house, he was willing to do it. He made it a habit to take off his shoes as soon as he got home, switched to unscented laundry products, used nonsolvent cleaning supplies, threw out his air fresheners and nonstick pans, and installed high-quality air filters in his heating and air-conditioning system.

Sure enough, several weeks after he cleaned house, he stopped getting hives and realized he'd lost most of those 15 extra pounds without ever thinking about it or doing anything other than cleaning the toxins out of his house.

This was an amazing thing for him, and he soon became one of my biggest word-of-mouth marketers. After six months, he'd lost all 15 pounds and had signed up for his first triathlon in five years. Unless he suddenly started eating far too many calories or reintroduced toxins into his life, he could expect to stay at a stable, healthy weight.

A House Full of Toxins

You can't always avoid the environmental toxins outside of your home such as exhaust fumes and contaminants produced by factories and power plants if you live in or near a city, or agricultural pollution if you live in a rural area. And you may not have much control over the toxins in your workplace either. Your industry may be hazardous by nature, or the building you work in may be so new that it's practically hermetically sealed, keeping the same air circulating—germs, toxins, and all. With the new modular cubicle office landscapes that feature carpeted floors and partitions, along with new pressboard-laminated furniture, computers, fax machines, and copiers, the levels of formaldehyde, ozone, and solvents are extremely high in many buildings. This has led to a rash of "sick buildings," with many workers getting sick building syndrome. With all of that going on outside of your home, it's more important than ever for your living space to be as clean and green as possible. But most homes are just the opposite, filled with toxins and toxic fumes that are locked in by airtight energy-efficient building techniques.

As a result of the oil shortage of the 1970s, building methods called for a cutback on the exchange of inside and outside air so that less energy would be needed to maintain a home's internal temperature. As a consequence, these homes retain more of the gases given off by things like carpeting than less airtight homes do.

At the same time, there has been a tremendous increase in the use of solvent-containing compounds in building materials, fabrics, and home furnishings. It's a truly vicious circle, isn't it? The use of

---

Indoor Air Pollutants

Combustion by-products from:
- Fireplaces
- Smoking
- Candles
- Stoves
- Water heaters
- Furnaces
- Attached garages

Solvents (volatile organic compounds) from:
- Paint
- Glue
- Carpeting
- Household cleaners
- Perfumes

Dusts and particulates from:
- Molds
- Cigarette smoke
- Infectious agents
- Animal dander
- Chemicals from indoor building supplies
- Pesticides

standard plywood gave way to the use of less-costly chipboard that contains more formaldehyde and solvents. Plywood laminate beams with higher formaldehyde content have replaced real wood beams. Flooring has gone from hardwood to plywood with pad and carpeting, all of which off-gas, releasing solvents and plastics. And recently, an estimated 100,000 new and remodeled homes in the United States have incorporated drywall board from China that's off-gassing toxic sulfur fumes into the homes.

The 1970s also saw changes in home-furnishing materials that put solvents into indoor air. Polyurethane foam and polyester fiberfill replaced traditional cotton batting upholstery fillers in sofas and chairs, and synthetic fabrics replaced cotton, rayon, and silk in draperies and upholstery. The upholstery fabrics themselves contain formaldehyde to prevent them from wrinkling. Plastic items, which off-gas plasticizers known as phthalates, are now found throughout the home. The rise of the home office, complete with computer, fax machine, and copier, has also increased the amounts of ozone, plastics, and other solvents present in our homes. Add paints, glues, gas heating and appliances, attached garages, biological contaminants of molds and bacteria, and storage of paints, paint thinner, gasoline, pesticides, and herbicides to the mix and the result is a very toxic home environment.

The worst offender by far is smoking, which leaves behind solvents, combustion byproducts, heavy metals, and cancer-causing chemicals for you to breathe in. So the biggest change anyone could make would be to quit smoking, or at the very least quit smoking indoors. This is especially bad for children, who retain up to 15 times the amount of airborne pollutants from smoking that adults do, and children have smaller bodies in which to try to disperse them.

The next most potent exposures at home come from new paint, new carpeting, new cabinetry, and new furniture. The formaldehyde and other compounds in these materials can take from five to fifteen years to finish off-gassing. And when the process finally runs its course, chances are somebody will decide that the carpet's starting to look worn and replace it, starting the cycle all over.

Top Ten Ways to Minimize Your Exposure to Solvents

1. Declare your home a shoe-free zone. Taking off your shoes before you enter your living space is one of the most effective ways to avoid bringing multiple outdoor toxins into your home.
2. Don't smoke or permit smoking inside your home or car.
3. Use an organic dry cleaner or air out dry cleaning in your garage, on your porch, or in your car trunk for a week before bringing it into the house.
4. Use unscented laundry detergent and fabric softener.
5. Don't use air fresheners that contain solvents.
6. Replace your furnace filters every six weeks with high-quality pleated filters rated a minimum efficiency reporting value (MERV) of 7–9. They cost more but are well worth it.
7. Buy an air purifier that has both charcoal and high-efficiency particulate air (HEPA) filters for your bedroom. The best are IQAir and Blueair. Make sure you get one that purifies enough cubic feet of air per minute (CFM) to clear the air in your bedroom at least once every thirty minutes.
8. Replace your carpet with tile flooring or prefinished real wood flooring. (Do not use the flooring made of pressboard with a thin veneer of wood on top. The pressed wood is held together with nasty chemicals that will be off-gassing into your indoor air for years to come.)
9. Make sure there isn't mold growth anywhere in your home, and if there is, be sure it's taken care of completely (not just hidden away) by a licensed contractor who can do a proper job of remediation.
10. Install a chlorine filter on your showerhead.

I know it's hard to believe that everyday household items could harbor such dangers to our health. Your home is supposed to be a haven from all of that. You can *make* it a haven by taking a close look at what's taken up residence in your house and evicting anything that doesn't measure up.

Still not convinced that such drastic measures are required? Read on. In 1985, the Total Exposure Assessment Methodology (TEAM) study by the EPA changed the way we look at indoor air quality (IAQ). The study showed that the greatest personal exposure to solvents comes from air in the home, not from outside air, as we used to think.

The study looked for the presence of twenty solvents in indoor air, outdoor air, breath, and personal air (the air that surrounds us as individuals) in 355 people in Elizabeth and Bayonne, New Jersey, where there are lots of chemical plants. Personal air was tested by attaching sampling cartridges to the study participants' clothing. The samples revealed very high levels of exposure to eleven solvents—sometimes 10 times higher than outdoor-air concentrations. The biggest source of these personal exposures was indoor air, which showed much higher levels of solvents, especially at night, than what was measured in the backyards of the same homes in the same time frame.

The Volatile Organic Compounds Consistently Found in Breath Samples in the TEAM Study
Chloroform
1,1,1-trichloroethane
Benzene
Carbon tetrachloride
Trichloroethylene
Tetrachloroethylene
Styrene
m,p-dichlorobenzene
Ethylbenzene
o-xylene
m,p-xylene

Since both the Elizabeth and the Bayonne areas are home to chemical plants, you might assume that outdoor chemicals would be responsible for the presence of most of the indoor chemicals found. But that wasn't the case. The compounds found most commonly were paradichlorobenzene (from mothballs and deodorants), styrene (plastics, foam rubber, insulation, and paints), tetrachloroethylene (dry cleaning), vinylidene chloride and xylene (paints), and benzene, ethylbenzene, and xylene (gasoline and cigarette smoke). And higher levels of benzene, xylene, and tetrachloroethylene were recorded after study participants had been to gas stations or dry cleaners. Levels were also higher in smokers than in nonsmokers.

The chloroform levels found were probably due to chlorine that all cities use as a disinfectant in water supplies. A Texas study showed

Our Most Common Daily Sources of Toxin Exposure

DAILY ACTIVITIES ASSOCIATED WITH HIGH PERSONAL EXPOSURE TO TOXIC COMPOUNDS

Activity	Volatile Organic Compound
Smoking	Benzene, xylene, styrene, ethylbenzene
Visiting the service station	Benzene
Driving	Benzene
Visiting the dry cleaner	Tetrachloroethylene
Working at a chemical plant	Ethylbenzene, styrene, xylene
Painting	Ethylbenzene, styrene, xylene
Working in a plastics plant	Ethylbenzene, styrene, xylene

HOME PRODUCTS ASSOCIATED WITH HIGH PERSONAL EXPOSURE TO TOXIC COMPOUNDS

Product	Volatile Organic Compound
Mothballs, deodorants	Paradichlorobenzene
Plastics, foam rubber	Styrene
Insulation	Styrene
Dry cleaning	Tetrachloroethylene
Paints	Vinylidene chloride, styrene, xylene
Gasoline	Benzene, ethylbenzene, xylene
Tap water	Chloroform, bromodichloromethane
Cigarettes	Benzene (twice nonsmokers' level), styrene

that levels of trihalomethanes—environmental pollutants such as chloroform that are produced when chlorine disinfectants combine with other materials in the water—rose significantly in the blood of women tested after they'd showered. For years, chloroform was used to anesthetize people before surgery because its effects on brain function are so potent. And here you thought it was just the hot water that made a shower so relaxing!

When the TEAM researchers expanded their study to include homes in North Carolina and North Dakota, their findings mirrored what they'd found in New Jersey: there was no correlation between outdoor pollutant sources and indoor levels. The indoor toxins all came from indoor sources. Let that roll around in your brain for a minute.

The researchers then decided to see whether certain activities would increase a person's exposure to these toxic compounds. To gauge this, they got seven volunteers to wear personal-exposure cartridges and keep track of what they did every day. The highest solvent exposures were associated with using deodorizers (air fresheners) in the home or workplace, washing clothes and dishes, visiting the dry cleaner's, smoking, painting and using paint remover, and working in scientific laboratories.

Previous studies that had looked at more than eight hundred people found the same thing. They all reported that each of the forty or more solvents studied were found in higher concentrations indoors than outdoors, often ten times higher. The sources of these compounds included building materials, furnishings, dry-cleaned clothes, cigarettes, gasoline, cleansers, moth crystals, hot showers, and printed materials.

The EPA followed up the TEAM studies with the nonoccupational pesticide exposure study (NOPES) to look for pesticide exposure. They chose two areas with relatively little agricultural pesticide use: the neighboring cities of Springfield and Chicopee, Massachusetts, and Jacksonville, Florida, where household pesticide use was relatively high. They found that concentrations of pesticides tended to be high in the summer, lower in the spring, and lowest in the winter. Indoor and personal air was usually much more toxic than outdoor air, just as the TEAM study had found with solvents.

The study also looked at the number of pesticides in the carpeting of nine homes in Jacksonville and found an average of twelve in the carpet dust (compared with an average of 7.5 in the air samples of the same residences). As the authors of the study pointed out, those most likely to be exposed to carpet-dust pesticides are infants and toddlers, who may ingest them when they put hands, toys, and other objects into their mouths. A Seattle study found that after application of the very toxic organophosphate pesticide chlorpyrifos, the levels in the infants' breathing zones—close to the floor—were higher than those in the adult breathing zones. The infants' exposure levels were 1.2 to 5.2 times greater than the level thought to be safe (the no-observable-effect level).

Clearly, we're not safe even in our own homes. To truly clean up the toxins in your body, you need to eliminate the toxins you're exposed to every day in your home. The dangers lurk in every room, but most are simple to remove or replace once you know what you're looking for and where to find it. And make no mistake—your home's "diet" will be at least as important in maintaining your weight loss as cutting the toxins out of what you eat.

If It Looks Clean and Smells Clean, It May Be Toxic

Don't be fooled by the look or artificial scent of "clean." Here are some of the worst offenders.

Air Fresheners

Some air fresheners contain a rogues' gallery of solvents that lead to respiratory troubles in animals. In one study, exposing mice to a commercially available freshener for an hour resulted in increased sensory and pulmonary irritation, difficulty breathing, and abnormal behavior. What does this mean for you? Air fresheners release chemicals in the form of tiny particles that you breathe in, and the next thing you know they're in your bloodstream. Plug-in air fresheners are even worse, since they emit these particles throughout the day. If you look at a can of air freshener at the grocery store, the label will probably include a carefully worded drug-abuse warning. That's because they're loaded with toluene, which, besides causing respiratory problems, is a potent toxin to the brain. Anything we breathe in goes right into the bloodstream and gets delivered throughout the body. Even diesel-exhaust soot has been found in the mitochondria of brain cells.

Soaps, Fragrances, and Perfumes

Fragrance-laden fabric softeners have been found to emit several known respiratory irritants. When mice were exposed to them (dryer sheets were put in their cages), they developed nose and lung sensitivity 23 percent to 49 percent of the time. They also experienced a restriction of their breathing anywhere from 6 percent to 32 percent of the time. After I mentioned these studies to Sal—and after he worked through his astonishment—things started making sense to him. He was beginning to understand why he felt as if he were under assault by his very environment.

What a way to live. We add fabric softener to our wash to make our clothes soft and smell good, and when we wear those clothes—as soft and fresh smelling as they may be—they restrict our breathing. Obviously, that clean-clothes smell isn't as clean as we thought. In fact, no matter how much we might enjoy a particular scent or perfume, there's nothing healthier than plain, old-fashioned fresh air. This is true for everyone but especially so for people with asthma, as another study showed. When asthma sufferers were exposed to perfumes from magazine scent strips, their breathing became much more difficult. More than 20 percent of them also experienced chest tightness and wheezing. Not exactly what you want to get out of reading a magazine or picking up a greeting card at a potpourri-scented gift shop. If you walk into a shop and feel a catch in your throat, your nose starts to tingle or itch, or your eyes start to water, your body's toxin-detection system is sending you an alert. So turn around and walk out.

One of the most interesting studies on the effects of the use of perfume looked at women with gynecological problems. The two compounds musk xylene (MX) and musk ketone (MK) are the most common chemical bases for the scents in perfumes, and they were found, respectively, in 95 percent and 85 percent of the women who were referred to a German hospital for a workup on their female hormones. Women who reported using perfumes four times a week or more showed significantly higher levels of MK than women who didn't use perfumes as often. The higher the levels of musk ketones in the blood, the more these young women complained of intense symptoms of premenstrual syndrome (PMS). Women with higher MX levels had lower estrogen and progesterone levels, more incidence of poorly functioning ovaries and, of course, more infertility. Women who were unable to conceive had significantly higher MX levels than women who had been pregnant once. The researchers also noted that women who had experienced one or more miscarriages consistently had higher levels of MX in their blood.

So the ultimate price of splashing on perfume that's supposed to make you feel sexy and help attract your perfect mate is a bad case of PMS, infertility, and possible miscarriage.

Cosmetics

The Environmental Working Group (EWG) recently found sixteen chemicals commonly used as preservatives for cosmetics and body-care products in blood and urine samples from twenty girls ages fourteen to nineteen. All of the chemicals came from bad families: phthalates (plasticizers), triclosans (commonly used chemicals that kill bacteria and other small organisms), parabens (chemicals used to kill microbes), and musk (the basic fragrance compounds we've just discussed). All have been linked to health problems such as cancer and hormone disruption. These were the first tests of paraben exposure among teens, and they indicate that young women are widely exposed to them. Two of the parabens, methylparaben and propylparaben, were found in every girl tested.

New research suggests that teens may be especially sensitive to hormone disruptors, like the ones in cosmetics, given the intricate network of hormonal signals that's leading them from childhood to adulthood. Talk about bad timing—during this period of vulnerability, adolescent girls experiment with more and more body-care products. In the EWG study, teen study participants used an average of nearly seventeen personal-care products a day, while the average adult woman uses just twelve. In the EWG study, girls with the highest

COMMON CHEMICALS FOUND IN FRAGRANCE PRODUCTS

Chemical	Odor Description	Possible Health Effects*
acetone	n/a	Skin, eye, and mucosa irritation; headache; nausea; drowsiness
benzaldehyde	Strong, sharp, sweet bitter, almond, cherry	Respiratory irritation; CNS depression; liver damage; dermatitis
benzyl acetate	Sweet, floral, fruity fresh	Skin, eye, and respiratory tract irritation; decrease in blood pressure and depth of respiration; increase in cardiac rate
benzyl alcohol	Light, floral, rose	Skin, eye, and respiratory tract irritation; delayed lung injury; GI disturbances; nausea; headache; dizziness
camphor	Camphor, minty, phenolic, woody	Burning sensation; coughing; wheezing; laryngitis; shortness of breath; headache; severe irritation of the mucosa, upper respiratory tract, eyes, and skin; flickering, darkening or veiling of vision; noises in the ears; weakness; feeling of warmth; CNS depression; difficulty breathing
1,8-cineole	Eucalyptus, mint, herbal, rosemary	Epigastric burning; nausea; vomiting; vertigo; ataxia; muscle weakness; stupor; pallor
ethanol	n/a	Skin and eye irritation; headache; nausea
ethyl acetate	Dry, fruity, musty pineapple	Headache; nausea; vomiting; narcosis
limonene	Lemon	Skin irritation and sensitization; eye irritation and damage; dizziness; rapid and shallow breathing; tachycardia; bronchial irritation; unconsciousness; convulsions
methylene chloride	n/a	Eye and respiratory tract irritation; headache; dizziness; stupor; nausea; vomiting; paresthesias of the extremities; skin inflammation; skin burns; unconsciousness
α-pinene	Fresh, sweet, pine, earthy, woody	Palpitations; dizziness; nervous disturbances; chest pain; bronchitis; benign skin tumors

Source: Wallace LA, Nelson WC, Pelizzari E, Raymer JH, Thomas KW. Identification of polar volatile organic compounds in consumer products and common microenvironments. Proceedings of Air & Waste Management Association 84th Annual Meeting and Exhibition, June 16–21, 1991, Vancouver, British Columbia.

*Some health effects may occur as a result of chronic or high level exposures to the chemical.

Abbreviations: CNS, central nervous system; GI, gastrointestinal.

levels of chemicals had the most problems with their menstrual cycles, including exceedingly painful periods.

Unfortunately, federal health statutes don't require companies to test personal-care products for safety before they're sold. As a result, few companies go to that effort. More than a third of all personal-care products include at least one ingredient linked to cancer, according to the EWG's Skin Deep database (which, by the way, is an indispensable source of information that you should consult before you make any cosmetics purchase—www.cosmeticsdatabase.org). To avoid this exposure, use natural products, mostly organic. You've probably heard it said, but it bears repeating: if you can't eat it, don't put it on your skin. You don't want to eat pesticides or foods that have been depleted of their nutrients, so don't put pesticides or highly processed ingredients on your skin. If you're going to eat 6 pounds of lipstick in your lifetime, as the average woman does, stick to ones that aren't going to hurt you.

What to Avoid in Cosmetics

If you find any of these on ingredient lists, evict the products from your medicine cabinet:

- Antibacterial compounds. Substances such as triclosan and chlorphenesin aren't biodegradable and may contribute to the rising number of bacteria that are resistant to antibiotics. Also, triclosan is a chlorinated antimicrobial agent and may bioaccumulate in us just like any chlorinated pesticide. We don't have documentation on this, but it would be best to err on the side of caution.
- Endocrine disrupters. Ingredients such as oxybenzone and methoxycinnamate are known endocrine disrupters and lurk in sunscreens. Look for sunscreens with titanium dioxide and zinc oxide instead.
- MEA/DEA/TEA. Used as foaming agents and stabilizers and for adjusting cosmetics' pH levels, these ammonia compounds can cause allergic reactions, eye irritation, and dry skin and hair.
- Parabens. These antimicrobial chemicals are used as preservatives and, like phthalates, can also disrupt hormones, according

to the EPA. But the antiparaben push seems to be gaining ground, with paraben-free stickers appearing on products such as lotions, soaps, deodorants, and toothpastes.

- Petrochemicals. Petroleum-based ingredients such as petrolatum, mineral oil, and paraffin (derived from nonrenewable sources) prevent the skin from breathing and can clog pores.
- Sulfates. These detergents are what makes soaps and shampoos lather up so nicely. Responsible for acid rain, they come from petroleum or vegetable oils that can be contaminated with pesticides, and they can irritate eyes and skin.
- Synthetic colors. Made from coal tar, these can contain heavy-metal salts (formed when nasty heavy metals such as cadmium bind with minerals). They're absorbed through the skin and can be toxic to the entire body. Animal studies have shown that most cause cancer. Beware of FD&C or D&C on the label.
- Synthetic fragrances. They often contain phthalates, plasticizers that are also used to stabilize fragrances and disrupt the endocrine (hormone) system and may alter genital development. Although industrial-chemical law considers phthalates to be toxic substances, the FDA doesn't regulate their use in body care, so manufacturers are free to mask their presence with the vague terms *fragrance* and *parfum* and claim that the ingredients are trade secrets. Unless the label says a fragrance is derived from essential oils or doesn't include phthalates, don't buy it if you don't know what's in it.
- Synthetic polymers. These make lotions nice and smooth, but they also make toxins during the manufacturing process.
- Ureas. These preservatives release tiny amounts of formaldehyde and are a leading cause of contact dermatitis. Their use is banned or restricted in other countries. If you see the terms *diazolidinyl urea, imidazolidinyl urea, DMDM, hydantoin,* or *sodium hydroxymethylglycinate* on the label, pass.
- 1,4-dioxane. This carcinogen is created when petroleum-derived ethylene oxide is part of the manufacturing process; it's added to fatty acids to make them more water soluble, a process known as ethoxylation. Companies aren't required to list 1,4-dioxane as an ingredient, since it's a byproduct of manufacturing, so look

for the USDA Organic seal—products bearing the seal don't include ethoxylated compounds. And steer clear of these ingredients: sodium myreth sulfate, ammonium laureth sulfate, oleth, cetearath, and polyethylene glycol (PEG) compounds, including polyoxyethylene and phenoxyethanol. Here's a memory aid: *eth* usually means "ethoxylated." And if you can't remember that, just remember that *eth* sounds like *meth*. Definitely somewhere you don't want to go.

After pitching all of the products that don't make the cut, be sure to check the EWG's cosmetics database to find out what you can safely restock your medicine cabinet with.

Understanding Packaging Symbols

The symbols on the packaging let you know if what you're buying is organic or at least genuinely natural. Here's what to look for:

Natural Certifications
- The Natural Seal. Granted by the Natural Products Association, this seal applies to products made up of at least 95 percent natural ingredients. And any synthetic ingredients that are used aren't linked to health risks.
- Premium Body Care. This seal applies to more than 1,200 items sold at Whole Foods stores. Products must stick to ingredients that are "as close to nature and as minimally processed as possible," have minimal effect on the environment, and aren't likely to cause skin irritations or allergies.
- Certified Natural Cosmetics. The BDIH, a German association of companies that produce and sell medicine, health products, dietary supplements, and skin-care products, grants this seal to companies that use plant ingredients whenever possible and avoid synthetic colors and fragrances, silicone, paraffin, and other petroleum products.

Organic Certifications
- USDA. The USDA organic seal applies to lotions, soaps, and shampoos that consist of at least 95 percent organic ingredients according to agricultural standards.

- NSF International. The NSF mark reveals how organic a product is—what percentage consists of organic ingredients—and the standards prohibit the use of ingredients and processes that aren't organic, including ethoxylated ingredients and synthetic fragrances.
- Organic Standard. The British Soil Association's Organic Standard symbol applies to products made up of at least 95 percent organic ingredients. It also has labels for products that are at least 70 percent organic (if the rest of the ingredients have been deemed safe for human and marine life).
- Ecocert. A label from the European-based organic-certification organization means that 95 percent of a product's ingredients are natural or "from natural origin." The label also means that genetically modified organisms, mineral oil, synthetic fragrance, ethoxylation, parabens, and animal testing have not been involved.

Dry Cleaning

Everybody loves to have their favorite clothing professionally cleaned and pressed. Many people visit a dry cleaner on a regular basis. But while it's great to have our clothes look impeccable, what dry cleaning brings to our lungs and our homes isn't so great. The solvents used to dry-clean clothes are quite potent, and there are stringent rules about how they can be disposed of because of their adverse effects on the environment. And bringing freshly dry-cleaned clothes into the home increases the detectable levels of those same nasty dry-cleaning solvents in the indoor air. Elevated levels of one of them—tetrachloroethylene—were found in one study after newly cleaned clothing was brought into the house, and they remained elevated for forty-eight hours. The study also found that the levels of this potent neurotoxin rose even higher with each additional garment that was brought into the house. And where do we typically put freshly dry-cleaned clothing? In the closet of the bedroom, the room where we spend the most time every day. This ensures that while we're sleeping, we'll be breathing in potent toxins. Was that your plan?

As for dry cleaners themselves, they can't seem to leave their work at the office. Elevated levels of the solvent trichloroethylene were found in their homes, too, having been carried in on their clothes and in their lungs and bloodstreams. They would have continued to exhale the solvent into their homes for hours after being at the shop because it can last that long in the bloodstream.

Carpeting

Carpeting is a perfect example of a home improvement that seems like a wonderful idea for transforming a room but turns out to be one of the most effective ways to poison a room. While the carpet industry is spending a lot of money to make you think all of the best houses have carpet, my advice is to be strong and resist this hard sell. I half-jokingly tell my patients that the only reason to get wall-to-wall carpeting is if they have a bug problem in their home—put in wall-to-wall and the toxic chemicals will kill the bugs as handily as any exterminator could. One little problem, though: the house isn't fit to live in as long as the carpet's in there.

Carpeting can be a big factor in the indoor emission of solvents and a great place for pesticide residues to hide out. When the EPA investigated the cause of toxicity at its own headquarters in 1988, it found that many of the elevated solvent levels were caused by new carpeting, and it ended up removing 27,000 square yards of it to make the building less sick.

A partial list of the chemicals found in carpeting is presented below. Many of the compounds, including benzene, xylene, and styrene, are known neurotoxins. When Anderson Laboratories tested carpet for its effects on the nervous system, mice were exposed to air that had been blown over carpet samples. Neurotoxicity—sometimes fatal—was found in more than 90 percent of the four hundred mice tested.

A Partial List of Chemicals in Carpets

Acetonitrile	Diphenyl ether
Azulene	Dodecane
Benzene	Ethylzylene
Biphenyl	5-methyltridecane
Butadiene	Formaldehyde
Cyclopentadiene-ethenyl-2-ethylene	4-phenylcyclohexane
	Hexadecanol

Hexamethylene triamine   1,2,3-trimethylbenzene
Isocyanates   Oxarium
Methacrylic acid   Phthalic acid esters
Methyl methacrylate   Polyacrylates
Octadecenyl amine   Styrene
1-chloronaphthalene   Tetradecene
1-ethyl-3-methylbenzene   Trichloroethylene (TCE)
1,4-dihydroxyacenophthene   Toluene
1-h-indene   2-butyloctanol-1
1-methylnaphthalene   2-methylnaphthalene
1-methyl-3-propylbenzene   2,3,7-trimethyldecane
1-methyl-4-tridecene   Undecane, 2,6-dimethyl
1,2,4-trimethylbenzene   Xylene
1,3,5-cycloheptatriene

Obviously, you'd have to be a chemistry major to identify all of these chemicals, but even those of us who aren't can make an educated guess that many of these compounds probably aren't good for us and should be avoided. And we would be correct.

Not all of these polysyllabic compounds are in all carpeting. Different types of carpet will give off different chemicals. Testing of rubber-backed carpet, for example, showed high emission levels of styrene and 4-phenylcyclohexene (4-PCH), which create that new carpet smell, while carpet with a polyvinyl chloride backing emitted a toxic cloud of formaldehyde, vinyl acetate, isooctane, 1,2-propanediol, and 2-ethyl-1-hexanol. All you need to know about these compounds is that there's nothing good about breathing them in.

A study in Swedish primary schools showed that chronic sick building syndrome was related to the presence of wall-to-wall carpeting. Once the carpet was removed, the number of reported symptoms declined. Another study found that among the household items linked to increased asthma rates, wall-to-wall carpeting was one of the main culprits. Despite it all, read real estate ads and you'll see that wall-to-wall carpeting is a selling point, particularly in bedrooms and living rooms—where most people spend the most time at home.

Carpet is also a magnet for dirt, toxic and nontoxic chemicals, and mold spores. If you've ever pulled up carpeting in your home, you know just how dirty it really is. There's a truly amazing amount of fine dirt on the floor under a carpet, and believe it or not, there's much more in the carpet itself. So you can pretty much count on any toxins that you track in or release into your home to get stuck in the carpeting and stay there. Studies have even found lead in carpets. Lead can come from old paint (in homes painted before 1978), the burning of metal-wicked (slow-burning) candles, and vinyl miniblinds. Lead can also be present in homes near busy roadways, having absorbed it during the many years when leaded gasoline was being used. No matter what the source, lead is released as a very fine dust that we can breathe in and that can land on carpeting, fabric, and other surfaces. Surprisingly, carpet and surfaces—rather than old paint—are the main avenues of elevated lead levels in toddlers' blood. Unfortunately, normal cleaning is not effective in reducing lead and pesticide levels in old carpets and upholstered furniture. If your furnishings are contaminated, it's time to buy new ones.

I've had more than one family come to me with health problems that were directly related to carpeting in their homes. Among the many tough sells I confront when dealing with my patients is getting them to rip out new carpet that they just spent thousands of dollars on. Often, the installation of new wall-to-wall carpeting is a project that's been months or years in the planning. And now they come to me and I tell them to get rid of it? Well, let's just say some of them don't come back for a while.

Of course people want to be healthy, and if they have children, they want to provide them with a healthy environment. But the idea that their soft, plush carpeting is a silent toxic stalker can seem inconceivable to some parents. Shaun's parents were such a case. Shaun was ten years old and suffered from debilitating allergies and migraines. He was also experiencing fatigue that was quite uncommon for a ten-year-old. After I gathered a history and pieced together all of the facts, the timing made it very clear to me that the problem was the carpeting his parents had just installed.

When I said this, they looked at me as if I'd grown another head or maybe sprouted horns. I'm sure they thought I was a quack or an extremist at best. Long story short, I didn't see them again for a year. When they finally returned, Shaun's condition was worse than before. In the interim, they'd gone to several other naturopathic and allopathic physicians who were unable to help. I retook Shaun's case and came to the same conclusion as before: take the carpet out! Even though the carpet had now become even more expensive—figuring in all of those other medical bills—they were still reluctant and wanted proof. When I suggested that Shaun spend some time away from home, they arranged for him to spend two weeks at his grandmother's house, which didn't have carpeting. When Shaun's headaches and fatigue lifted within days of being there, they finally believed me and had the carpet removed. Once it was gone, the toxins that had been plaguing Shaun were gone, too. Within days, his symptoms disappeared, and he went back to being a happy, healthy eleven-year-old boy again.

I'm sure by now you've figured out that if you stopped by my house, you wouldn't have to worry about spilling anything on the carpet. Kelly and I are both very grateful that we learned all of this before we had our little girl. It's wonderful to see her crawling around on a clean floor and know that being carpet free is keeping her from building up her toxic burden. When I think about all of the babies who are crawling around on carpets that are outgassing chemicals toxic to their nervous and immune systems, I fear for the next generation.

Indoor Building Materials

Sometimes the toxins permeating your home are coming from inside the walls, beneath your floorboards, and above your ceilings—places that you can't even see. Many building materials used in home construction contain formaldehyde, solvents, glues, and other resins. All of these emit chemicals into the air of the home for years. Even plastic plays a role in our home air pollution. Contractors are turning to it more and more because it makes for inexpensive, easy-to-clean surfaces for kitchen walls and floors and in bathrooms and areas where kids play. Unfortunately, it also emits polyvinyl chloride and other plasticizers, including phthalates, into the air. A study in Finland revealed that the presence of plastic can dramatically increase the incidence of respiratory ailments in children. Use linoleum, stone, or tile instead.

VOLATILE ORGANIC COMPOUNDS EMITTED BY BUILDING MATERIALS AND INTERIOR FURNISHINGS

Source	Pollutant Emitted
Adhesives	Alcohols, benzene, formaldehyde, terpenes, xylenes
Caulking compounds	Alcohols, benzene, formaldehyde, methylketone, xylenes
Carpeting	Formaldehyde, 4-methylbenzene, styrene, stain-resistant chemicals, wrinkle-resistant chemicals
Particleboard	Alcohols, benzene, formaldehyde, terpenes, toluene
Vinyl tiles and flooring	Benzene, formaldehyde, methyl styrene, xylenes
Paints, stains, varnishes	Benzenes, formaldehyde, toluene

The table above gives you an idea of just how toxic modern building materials are.

If you're getting the sense that we can't win unless we live in grass huts, remember that it's a matter of degree. While we obviously can't do without all of the materials listed in the table, we can do without some of them, and every time you evict one of them from your home, your health benefits. Fortunately, many of these building products are now being made without such high levels of toxins. Check with your local building supplier for nontoxic alternatives. Just remember that if a product is labeled Green, that typically refers to its sustainability, not to its being less toxic, so get all of the facts before you buy.

Take a Toxin Tour of Your Home

Now that you know about the "double agents" that have been hindering your weight-loss efforts under the guise of providing comfort or convenience, it's time to take a walk around your house. No need to grab a trash bag just yet, though. In week two of the four-week plan, you'll have plenty of time to do the house cleaning. For now, just assess what you have in your home that's toxic and consider some of the options and tips I offer for cleaner and greener alternatives. We'll start with the rooms where you probably spend most of your time at home and work our way out to the garage and the yard.

Bedroom

You spend the largest chunk of any given day in this room, so the cleaner and greener you can make your bedroom, the better.

- Bed and bedding. I've worked with several patients whose toxic loads were pushed over the edge after they got new mattresses that contained lots of chemicals. Pillows and mattresses made of foam off-gas chemicals that you breathe in all night. And if your bedding has permanent press and stain-resistant properties, you probably have formaldehyde to thank for that. Instead, use mattresses and pads made of natural latex, and buy bedding made with natural fibers like cotton—they don't contain synthetics such as polyurethane, and they're naturally fire-resistant. At www.ewg.org/pbdefree, the EWG offers a database of bedding and other household furnishings that don't have flame retardants.
- Electrical cords. If you have a standard box spring with metal coils under your mattress, be sure there are no extension cords under the bed that are running your bedside clocks. Extension cords can contribute to electromagnetic charges in the coils. Avoid this extra stress on the body.
- Wall-to-wall carpeting. This modern luxury is loaded with chemicals that are toxic to both the immune system and the nervous system. In addition, it provides a hideout for toxins that have been circulating in the air.
- Waterbeds with pressboard frames. Many heated waterbeds are surrounded by 1½ inches of pressboard frame. The heat from the mattress dramatically increases the off-gassing of the chemicals in the pressboard and the finish on the wood.
- Air filters. You might as well be breathing the cleanest air possible while you sleep. Consider getting an air purifier that has both charcoal and HEPA filters. Make sure you get one that circulates enough cubic feet per minute (CFM) to clear the air in your bedroom at least once every thirty minutes. (I recommend IQAir and Blueair; see the resources at the back of this book.)

Determining Cubic Feet per Minute

Multiply the room's width by its length, and then multiply that figure by the height. That's the room's volume—the room's cubic footage. Multiply the volume by 2 (for two complete changes of all the air in the room in one hour). Finally, divide that figure by 60, and the result will be the number of cubic feet per minute that need to be cleaned.

Example:

Width (10 feet) x length (20 feet) = 200 square feet

200 square feet x height (8 feet) = 1,600 cubic feet

1,600 cubic feet x 2 (room air changes per hour) = 3,200 cubic feet per hour

3,200 cubic feet per hour / 60 minutes = 53.3 cubic feet per minute

Kitchen

- Cookware. Get rid of chemical-spewing nonstick pans. Ceramic titanium and porcelain-enameled cast iron are great alternatives.
- Canned food. Cut back on canned foods. The cans are lined with the plastic compound bisphenol A (BPA), which can leach into the foods. Look for organic brands that don't use bisphenol-A linings, such as Eden Foods.
- Plastic. Avoid microwaving food in contact with plastic containers or wraps. Store food in glass, stainless steel, porcelain, and plastics that are free of BPA and phthalates. Drink only from these, too. Don't wash plastic in the dishwasher, which can cause the plastic to leach endocrine disruptors. Throw out scratched or hazy-looking plastic containers, which are more prone to leaching. Don't put hot food in plastic or store food in plastic packaging for long periods of time.
- Plastic wrap. Choose plastic wrap made of polyethylene, such as Glad Cling Wrap and Handiwrap, rather than polyvinylidene chloride (Saran Wrap). Better yet, use waxed paper. And even

better still, use all of these as little as possible, and don't ever heat food in a microwave with these products.

- Water. To get the lead out, get a carbon water filter (it will also remove chlorine and other major toxic offenders). To go after toxins with smaller molecules, such as nitrates, trichloroethylene, and perchlorate, you'll need a more expensive reverse osmosis or granular-activated carbon filter. Finally, the most expensive option is a whole-house filter that goes after those smaller contaminants; this way you avoid drinking them and sharing your shower with them. All of these options are better for you than bottled water and far less expensive. And if you want to know exactly what toxins you're up against, check your water company's annual report on what's in your water. You can also have your water tested by a private lab; there's a list of them at www.epa.gov/safewater/labs, or call the EPA Safe Drinking Water Hotline, 800-426-4791. This step is especially advisable if you have a well.

- Dish washing. Buy dishwashing liquid that doesn't contain triclosan. And if the label says, Keep Away from Children, keep it away from you, too.

- Ventilation. Be sure that your stove vent fan is working well and that it's venting to the outside of your house. The fan will clear out smoke from cooking, other combustion fumes, and any natural gas vapors that may be present.

- Natural gas appliances. Many of my patients found that their health problems were directly linked to natural gas exposure in their homes. Environmentally aware physicians have long regarded natural gas appliances as a health hazard. Recently, women who use gas stoves for cooking were found to have a host of respiratory problems. They had a 200 percent greater risk of experiencing wheezing, a 232 percent greater risk of feeling short of breath, and a 260 percent greater risk of having asthma attacks. While we may love the way gas stoves are so responsive to our cooking needs, they're not exactly "a breath of fresh air" when it comes to health issues.

  If you have gas appliances (stove, oven, water heater, gas fireplace) and you can detect even a very faint odor of gas whenever you walk into your home or are in close range of these appliances, call your gas utility immediately. A gas leak is very serious.

Bathroom

- Bath/shower. Install chlorine filters in your showerhead.
- Personal hygiene products and cosmetics. Choose natural—organic whenever possible—and nontoxic personal products (soaps, shampoos, lotions, makeup) free of synthetic fragrances, parabens, and sodium lauryl sulfates.
- Cleaning products. Buy nonsolvent cleaning supplies (including tile cleaners and air fresheners) that are free of perfumes. Or make your own. Go to www.Care2.com to find easy recipes for nontoxic cleaning products that are cheaper than toxic commercial products and work just as well. The Web site www.lesstoxicguide.ca also offers recipes and lists nontoxic products by brand name.
- Ventilation. Have a good vent fan in the bathroom to clear the moisture out after a shower. Make sure the fan vents to the outside of the house, not into the attic space.
- Mold. Be sure there's no water damage in the bathroom. Check to make sure that the caulking around the shower pan is good. If mold is growing there, have a professional come in and check it. When caulking has been done improperly or gets old, it lets moisture through to the wallboard in back of the shower surround. The wallboard will then often act like a giant sponge and start to grow mold. You may not smell it, but it can be one of the most toxic presences in your home. Call in a professional to check it out and fix it immediately if mold is present. This goes for anywhere in the home. (If you're unsure whether there's mold in your home, contact a local indoor-air specialist who can test for mold. This may be the best investment you ever make.)
- Carpeting. There shouldn't be carpeting in the bathroom—unless you want mold. Use cotton throw rugs and bath mats that can be picked up and washed.

Living Room

- Carpeting and flooring. Consider replacing carpeting with hardwood, tile, or stone flooring. Don't get the hardwood that's made of pressboard with only a veneer of wood grain on the top—it will off-gas formaldehyde and other toxic compounds into your home for decades to come. Besides, good hardwood floors will increase the value of your home, as will good stone floors. If you stick with carpet, use a vacuum with a HEPA filter that traps dust and pollutants.
- Furniture. Get pressboard furniture out of your home. Many bookcases and entertainment centers are made of pressboard, with a nice wood veneer on the outside. This pressboard is basically made of sawdust glued together. Since the sawdust came from wood, these pieces may be advertised as being solid wood, but they aren't made from actual wood boards. These pressboard pieces can take five to fifteen years to give off all of the toxic chemicals they have to give.

Hall/Entryway

- Make your home a shoe-free zone by taking off your shoes as soon as you come inside. Shoes get covered with all of the pollutants outside, and what they track in is one of the biggest sources of contaminants in your home.

Laundry Room

- Washing. Use only unscented laundry detergent and fabric softener. If you must use bleach, opt for the chlorine-free version.
- Drying. When it comes to harmful household products, you can't get much more toxic than fabric sheets that include fragrance.

Basement

- Furnace and central air. Install high-quality pleated air filters (rated MERV 7–9) in your furnace and air-conditioning systems, and change them every month.
- Air ducts. Have a service come in and clean out the air ducts (but don't let them spray any chemicals inside the ducts when they're done). This will eliminate a load of chemical toxins that are attached to the dust in your home.

- Mold. Look for and eliminate mold and properly repair any water damage.

Garage

- Paints and cleaning and building supplies. Use only nontoxic paints and building materials for any household maintenance, repairs, remodeling, and construction.

Lawn and Garden

- Weeds. Pulling weeds with the proper weeding tools is relatively easy if you do it right after it rains or if you lightly water the area first. The more weeds you pull, the fewer herbicides you'll need, with the goal being zero.
- Insects. Learn natural methods of insect control. For example, you can plant marigolds to deter slugs, and you can put out a bat house to attract those ravenous mosquito eaters. Check out the Northwest Coalition for Alternatives to Pesticides online at www.pesticide.org for fact sheets that will give you other ideas. The Pesticide Action Network is another helpful resource. Its Web site, www.panna.org, lists nontoxic alternatives, and it has a searchable database of pesticide chemicals at pesticideinfo.org/Search_Chemicals.jsp.

Safe Weed Killer (safe for you—not for the weeds!)

1 gallon vinegar
1 cup salt
8 drops dish soap

Stir ingredients together in a bucket until well combined. Transfer to a container with a spray top. Spray on weeds. There's no need to wear a mask to protect yourself or to keep your kids or your pets off the lawn afterward. You'll probably have to spray the weeds a couple of times within a seven-day period. One of my patients brought this recipe to me, and I've shared it with many people. We've all found it to work well.

If your tour has left you feeling a little overwhelmed, take heart. Knowledge is power. And the key to lasting change is to tackle one toxin at a time, one room at a time. In the four-week plan, I'll provide you with checklists that make your cleaning steps easy.

Now that you know how to avoid eating and drinking toxins and how to get the nastiest ones out of your home, it's time to learn how to get the nastiest ones out of your body—as quickly and safely as possible.

PART THREE

Living Clean, Green, and Lean

CHAPTER 7

The Clean, Green, and Lean Four-Week Plan

The most direct and lasting path to a new, lean you is getting clean and going green. Getting clean means "out with the bad." You'll begin lightening your toxic load and your weight by getting rid of all of the toxic food products in your pantry and refrigerator, and replacing them with nontoxic options that are healthier both for you and for the planet. Going green means "in with the good." For our purposes, *green* doesn't just mean organic or chemical free. It also means broccoli, green tea, and other good nutrients such as supplements. You'll be taking your clean and green steps in the same order as you learned about them in chapters 3 through 6, and within four weeks your world will be cleaner and greener and you'll be on your way to being lean for life.

Because toxic compounds are part of everyday living, losing weight by tackling the toxin problem can sound overwhelming. But I swear to you it's not. By making just a few simple changes a week, you can literally change your life. Getting rid of the bad and getting more of the good is the simplest way to lose weight and restore your body and mind to optimal health. It's the most natural way to live, and believe me, you'll begin to feel the positive changes almost immediately. Many of my patients begin to feel better as soon as they find out that there's a proven pathway out of the perpetual cycle of dieting and deprivation and into a lean lifestyle that makes them feel happy and inspired about their lives again.

The clean, green, and lean plan is a concrete week-by-week program that you can embrace as easily as you do the weekly routine you already follow. Over time, it will actually be easier than the way you're living now because you'll have an abundance of energy. When my patients reach this point, they realize how strongly their food cravings and fatigue were tied to their old toxic ways. With this plan, you won't need willpower to lose weight and keep it off, because now that you know what's poisoning you, you can move on to better choices. Rewarding yourself by eating something that tastes fantastic, feeds your mitochondria, and increases your energy will soon naturally replace energy-zapping candy, snacks, and soft drinks. Instead of feeding your toxic cravings, you'll be feeding your health and your happiness. Soon you'll find that living the clean, green, and lean life is as easy as getting out of bed in the morning (okay, as easy as getting into bed at night). And the process of giving your extra pounds the boot will be well under way.

As your toxic load drops and your health improves, you'll see the numbers on your scale go down. The two go hand in hand. And when you occasionally splurge on something a little less clean and green—like the fried fish and chips at your neighborhood pub or the cotton candy at the fair—you'll find that your body can handle a little of the "bad" from time to time. One of my colleagues at the Southwest College of Naturopathic Medicine eats sugar only on Sundays. Instead of giving up sugar entirely, something she doesn't want to do, she allows herself to indulge just one day a week. She's found this to be a perfect compromise that doesn't leave her feeling deprived. Many of my patients who use this sort of approach find that over time their taste buds actually change and they begin to prefer the taste of real maple syrup over the corn syrup brands, and they like using honey and agave nectar more than white refined sugar. Their tastes adjust and the pleasures of real food reveal themselves as nature intended, before chemicals started chipping away at their taste buds' sensitivity. So be prepared to prefer the healthier, less greasy potato chips to your old high-fat favorites. Remember, the clean, green, and lean lifestyle change is not about deprivation—it's about feeling great, losing weight, and looking better than you thought you could.

And now, prepare to amaze yourself. What you're holding in your hands is nothing less than your ticket to a cleaner, greener, and leaner you.

Setting Up the Plan

The best way to prepare yourself for the lifestyle change you've chosen to make is to get crystal clear about your intentions. What, specifically, do you want to achieve by detoxing and losing weight? How do you want to look? How do you want to feel? These are the types of questions that will clarify your intentions and empower you to stick with the plan for the duration.

Every New Year's Eve, my wife and I write out our intentions for the coming year and review the ones we wrote the previous year. We've seen the power of setting clear intentions and how rewarding it is to create beneficial changes in our lives. Having a clear vision of what you want to achieve aligns your mind and body with your goal. So set a clear, firm intention—or several intentions—for what you want to create in your life (the why and how will come later). This can include the clearing out of emotional toxins as well as physical ones.

Set Your Intentions

Intentions are statements that describe what you want to do. Remember that you're making a choice, so your intentions should reflect that by beginning with "I want to" or "I choose to" rather than "I have to" or "I need to." When you feel like you have to do something, it often creates a sense of desperation. So when you catch yourself thinking or saying "I have to," take a moment to remember that you don't have to do this at all, and as long as you allow yourself to play the victim game, you'll feel disempowered. So clean out the desperation and open up for inspiration.

Here are some examples that may help you while you're working on your own intentions:

- I want to release all of the restrictions (physical, mental, emotional, spiritual) that are keeping me from experiencing optimal health.
- I want to create an environment in my life that's toxin free and nurturing to every cell of my body.
- I choose to begin releasing all of the toxins (physical, mental, emotional, spiritual) from my body.
- I will make choices in my life every day that are self-loving and nurturing and that bring me to a greater state of health and well-being.

Don't worry if your intentions don't sound like these. You can change and refine them as you go along.

You may want to sit with your best friend or spouse, the one who's always straightforward with you, over a nice cup of green tea and talk about your intentions and why they're important to you. Doing this will probably help you refine them more quickly.

And now for the why: why do you want to become clean, green, and lean? "Do I really need a reason?" you might wonder. "Isn't the weight loss reason in itself?" The point is that by having a list of the benefits in your head, you may have more incentive and find it easier to make it happen. And this program is all about making it easy on you. So which is it—do you want more energy, to look better, to be able to keep up with the kids? Whatever your reasons, put them in writing.

Rate Your Physical Toxic Symptoms

Let's start with your physical health. Here's a table of the most common symptoms of toxicity and the most common health problems associated with toxins. Review the table and give a score to all that apply to you. Base the score on a scale of 1 to 10, with 10 being the most troubling.

TOXIC SYMPTOMS

Symptom or Health Problem	How It Rates Now (1–10)	Rating at Day 30	Rating at Day 60	Rating at Day 90	Rating at Day 180	Rating at Day 365
Fatigue						
Depression						
Brain fog						
Balance problems						
Poor memory						
Headaches						
Tremors						
Allergies						
Asthma						
Chemical sensitivity						
Diabetes						
Fibromyalgia						
Autoimmunity (rheumatoid arthritis, lupus, etc.)						
Infertility						
Chronic infections						
Bone marrow problems						
Parkinsonism						
Other						
Other						
Other						

Record Your Vital Statistics

You can also record your vitals below and some of the findings from your most recent laboratory testing. This can include measurement of toxic burden if you've been tested for it. In the top row, record the dates of the readings.

VITAL STATISTICS

Test	Reading as of:	Reading as of:	Reading as of:	Reading as of:	Reading as of:	Reading as of:
Weight						
Blood pressure						
Pulse at rest						
White blood cell count						
Red blood cell count						
Blood glucose						
Hemoglobin A1C						
Total cholesterol						
HDL cholesterol						
LDL cholesterol						
Triglycerides						
TSH						
Total chlorinated pesticides in serum						
Total PCBs in serum						
Total solvents in serum						

Assess Your Emotional Toxicity

It's been my experience that emotional toxins are linked with the physical toxins stored in your body. It seems that when people store a lot of emotional toxins (such as guilt, shame, fears, abuse, or some other type of major stress), their bodies will also store the physical toxins that are present. When the physical toxins are mobilized, the emotional toxins get churned up as well. Similarly, when people undergo counseling and begin to deal with their stored emotional toxins, their physical toxins also come rushing out.

When patients who have already done a lot of emotional and spiritual healing work come in to my clinic to do physical cleansing, I've been amazed at how quickly their bodies can dump those physical toxins. Because they've done the emotional work, their cleansing work goes quickly. They've laid the groundwork. On the other hand, those who refuse to even look at the possibility that they have emotional toxins progress very slowly with the mobilization of their physical toxins. So, being open to clearing both at the same time is very conducive to healing. The following chart is for those interested in exploring emotional toxins that may need to be addressed.

EXPLORING YOUR EMOTIONAL TOXINS

Emotional Toxin	How It Affects Me	How I Will Help Release This Trauma

Finding a great counselor can be a big help, as can support groups. For individual traumas, I've had excellent success using a couple of deceptively simple techniques. The easiest and most user-friendly is called the emotional freedom technique (EFT). You can use the technique on yourself, or you can look for a local therapist who uses the method. I even know of some physicians who use EFT to help their patients get over physical health problems. It's fantastic at helping to clear out the power of old traumas, fears, guilt, and beliefs that no longer serve you. You can find out about it by going to www.emofree.com.

Build Your Support Team

Finally, it's time to ask: how exactly will you reach the goals you've set? What else can help you succeed? For starters, how about a friend or a loved one who can support you in your decisions, cheer you on, and help to hold you accountable? The most successful changes typically come with the help of others, whether it's a workout partner or a personal coach. Having others help us, push us, cheer us, encourage us, and hold us accountable makes a big difference. So assemble your support team.

Questions to Help You Assemble Your Support Team
- How many team members do you want?
- What role will each person play?

Team Members to Consider
- A naturopathic or holistic physician to provide you with testing and medical support
- A massage therapist to help mobilize the toxins from your muscles
- A chiropractor to keep your skeletal structure in line as your body shifts and changes
- A counselor to help with clearing emotional toxins
- A handyman or woman to help with changes you make in your home
- A personal chef or someone to shop for groceries

MY CLEAN, GREEN, AND LEAN SUPPORT TEAM: CGL TEAM
[YOUR FIRST NAME HERE]

Name	What Role Will This Person Play on the Team?	Have You Asked Him or Her?	Has He or She Agreed?	Is He or She Going to Join You in Making the Changes?

You know yourself best, so as you look over the changes planned for the next week, watch for the places where your immediate reaction is "Oh, I can't do that" or "That's too hard." Then put a check mark by those changes so you don't forget which ones they are and ask yourself, "What or who can help me accomplish those changes with ease and grace?" If your intention is to change, allow the answer to show up, and include that person on your team.

Your team members may want to be more than just support for you—they may want to participate and join you in making these lifestyle changes. This will make it a true team effort, and you know that accomplishing goals as a team often works much better than individual efforts do.

Once you decide which players you want on your team, pick up the phone and schedule a meeting for the coming week.

Now let's get you started on your new lean life. You deserve it!

Week 1: Eating Clean, Green, and Lean

Your Goal: To identify and eliminate toxic foods from your menu and replace them with healthy alternatives that you enjoy just as much, if not more.

While it may not seem as if simply increasing your organic-food intake could make a difference in your health, it truly can. I recently received this letter from someone I've never met but who had read one of my articles about the benefits of eating organic foods:

Dear Dr. Crinnion:

Last September I started on a health journey that would lead me to where I am today. I started to get sick with an illness and started to get better when I found this article written by Walter J. Crinnion, N.D. I had lots of symptoms, starting with my left thumb twitching constantly for almost 3 months. It never stopped and then one night I went to bed and woke up with a heart rate so high I was vibrating. By the time I got to the ER (my heartrate) was almost 230. From that night on my heart rate sitting would be around 90 and, when standing without moving, would go over 150, and as I would walk it would climb sometimes up to 200. Just getting up to go to the bathroom or shower would leave me out of breath and exhausted. Playing with my kids was impossible and the heart palpitations were debilitating. I went to several local doctors, who all said that it was only ANXIETY and I needed some antidepressants. Finally, I went to Cleveland Heart Clinic and was diagnosed with Inappropriate Sinus Tachycardia (IST) and put on a beta blocker but was told that due to this being in the autonomic nervous system, the drugs probably would not do much good, so I should just try to live with it. So I tried to stay positive. I came back and found a pediatric cardiologist who treated adults with these conditions.

I started to get worse. My memory went, my vision was affected, along with my hearing. There were some days when I couldn't walk or lift my arms. I was falling apart. I went in for testing with an internist and he said it was most likely multiple sclerosis or rheumatoid arthritis or something along those lines. All my tests came back negative, including one they did for Lyme disease. I was also told it could be fibromyalgia with IST or that it was all in my head!!!! I always knew in my heart there was something causing all of this. I felt completely lost.

One night in bed I was online looking for information on chronic illness when I found an article regarding organic food by Dr. Crinnion. I read the statement "The more chronically ill people I see (in my practice), the bigger my organic garden gets"!!! At this point I didn't think about food or water and I was unaware of the many pesticides used. I read that article several times because it hit me like a ton of bricks and I walked down and threw out all the food in my kitchen and then next morning in an electric cart I bought 100% organic. I read other sites on organic and for the first time I felt some hope. After two weeks of eating organic something amazing happened, My heart rate when standing was normal and the palpitations were less, to the point where they were not affecting me—this all after two weeks. I called my doctor and he said if your heart rate has changed due to food changes, this is NOT true IST, it's from something else, which I had already known—just didn't know what.

Later the doctors wanted to put me on antibiotics, but I always came back to this article in my head, and if organic foods and what is NOT in them got rid of this horrible heart condition that I had lived with for 6 months, how could synthetic antibiotics and other things help me? The words I read I have taken with me through this journey. I can say in all honesty that this article saved my life and led me on the road to better health, better understanding, and I try to share these words with whoever will listen and those even who don't. I now take a lot of great things for my health, but most important are the organic food and clean water. I am now in "remission" from Lyme disease and will continue to live what I have learned because I do think it isn't a choice. Thank you for your article. It found me when I was drowning and lost and it was my light at the end of the tunnel!

MW, Front Royal, VA

If dramatic results like these are what you're looking for, it's time for action. And here are your action steps.

Get Clean

Grab a large trash bag, or, better yet, bring the whole can into the house. You probably have a lot to throw away.

1. Trash the Food That's Most Toxic

It would be best to clear out all of the nonorganic food, but at the very least get rid of the most toxic of the commercial varieties of foods. Take the following toxic ingredients off your menu:

Bisphenol A
Chlorinated pesticides
Flame retardants
Heavy metals
Inks
Organophosphate pesticides
Plastics
Polychlorinated biphenyls (PCBs)
Solvents

Your task is to go through your refrigerator and pantry, find the toxic foods, and throw them away. Start with the fruits and vegetables, whether they're fresh, frozen, canned, or dried, and then move on to dairy, meat, and fish.

FINDING THE MOST TOXIC FOODS

Food	In the House?	Action to Take with the Commercial Varieties in Your Home	Replacement
Peaches		Peel before eating	Buy organic
Apples		Peel before eating	Buy organic
Sweet bell peppers		Acid wash (see the box on page 44 in chapter 2)	Buy organic
Celery		Discard	Buy organic
Nectarines		Peel before eating	Buy organic
Strawberries		Discard—you cannot remove the pesticides by peeling or acid wash—sorry!	Buy organic. When fresh berries aren't available, remember to look for frozen organic berries, which are available year-round.
Cherries		Acid washing may help but often is not sufficient, so you may need to discard the cherries (if your mouth gets that chemical or metallic taste)	Buy organic
Pears		Peel before eating	Buy organic
Imported grapes		Acid washing may help but often is not sufficient, so you may need to discard the grapes (if your mouth gets that chemical or metallic taste)	Buy organic
Spinach		Discard	Buy organic
Lettuce		Discard	Buy organic
Potatoes		Peel before cooking	Buy organic
Nonorganic dairy products (milk, cheese, butter, ice cream) Nonorganic eggs Nonorganic beef		Discard	Buy organic

Food	In the House?	Action to Take with the Commercial Varieties in Your Home	Replacement
Atlantic salmon		Discard	Buy only Alaskan salmon–king, red, or silver
Canned tuna		Discard	Use canned Alaskan salmon
Swordfish		Discard	Use low-mercury fish instead
Shark		Discard	Use low-mercury fish instead
Orange roughy		Discard	Use low-mercury fish instead
Chilean sea bass		Discard	Use low-mercury fish instead
Lobster		Discard	Use low-mercury fish instead
Halibut		Discard	Use low-mercury fish instead
Snapper		Discard	Use low-mercury fish instead (listed under Go Green)

Check Your Oil

Are any of the oils you cook with in plastic containers? If so, they will leach plastic from the container and deliver a healthy (read "unhealthy") dose to you each time you use them. Be sure that your oils are in dark-colored glass containers that are kept in a dark, cool place. If your olive oil is kept next to the stove or above it, the heat has probably made it go rancid. You'll need to find a different place to keep the new bottle you'll get to replace it. Get rid of any rancid oils or oils in plastic containers.

Discard products that contain partially hydrogenated oils (PHOs). Trans fats, also listed on food labels as vegetable fat and vegetable shortening, are common food additives and are extremely unhealthy for you. They're commonly found in the processed foods in the inside aisles of the grocery store: chips, cookies, crackers, peanut butter, candies, and other snack foods.

2. Reduce and Remove Energy-Zapping Foods

Now it's time to clean your food pantry of the most common offender foods. These foods not only cause you to pack on weight, but also prevent your body from dumping toxins. Remove every item that contains:

Refined sugar
High-fructose corn syrup
White flour (ingredient labels often just list flour)

The worst offenders are the foods that have any of these as the first or second ingredient.

As for specifically eliminating sugars, first look at all of the labels. Is sugar one of the first three ingredients on any of them? If so, that makes it easy, and you can clear them out of your pantry and look for sugar-free replacements.

Hidden Sources of Sugar:

Is This on the Ingredient List?	In the House?
Corn syrup	
Dextrose	
Fructose	
High-fructose corn syrup	

If the label lists high-fructose corn syrup, throw it away and don't buy it again. Despite advertising that says this sweetener is natural, it's implicated in many current chronic health problems and has been found to be contaminated with the toxic heavy metal mercury.

Foods High in Sugar
Barbecue sauce
Cake
Candy
Cereals
Chocolate milk

Cookies
Doughnuts
Dried fruits
Flavored gelatins
Fruit-flavored yogurt and frozen yogurt
Fruit punch and fruit juices
Granola
Honey
Hot chocolate
Ice cream and ice cream bars
Jams and jellies
Juice bars
Lemonade
Muffins
Pies
Popsicles
Pudding
Soda—regular
Sweetened tea
Syrup
Tapioca
Toaster pastries

Also do the following:

- Dispose of all sweetened drinks. These drinks are the source of most of the sugars consumed in the United States. The average American's sugar load is about 100 pounds per year. Sugar is devastating to your health and your body, including your bones and your immune system.
- Avoid all carbonated sodas—including sugar free. Carbonated soft drinks leach calcium from your bones. The diet versions of soda are no better than those filled with sugar, and may be worse. The chemicals in diet soda and other sugar-free, artificially sweetened products are just that—chemicals. They are not food. They come from the same companies that brought us

DDT and told us it was a good thing. As chemicals, they're part of your total load of toxins, and they're very easy to avoid. So avoid them.

- Limit alcohol consumption to no more than once every two days. The healthiest of all alcoholic drinks are the deep red wines, which have antioxidants that are helpful to the body, and white wines, which can remove mercury stored in your brain. But be smart by being moderate.

- Limit full-strength fruit juices. Full-strength fruit juices provide a strong dose of fruit sugars. Typically, you can down a glass of orange juice, containing the juice of several oranges, within a minute or two. But it probably would have taken you all day or even a week to get around to eating that many oranges. When you eat the complete fruit, you also get the fibers from the fruit that slow the release of the fruit sugars into your bloodstream. These fibers are no longer present in a glass of juice. So your blood sugar will spike after you drink fruit juices, just as it does after you eat a piece of candy. One option is to water the juice down or mix it with sparkling water.

- Avoid all fast foods and deep-fried foods. If you still crave fast food, rent the movie *Super Size Me* so that you can see what actually happens to one person's health when he eats only fast food. Even some of the salads that are available at most fast-food restaurants appear to be about as healthy as the burgers. If you must have fast food for a treat, not a regular meal, keep it to no more than twice a month.

3. Uncover Your Weight-Loss Saboteurs

Many people have adverse reactions to a number of foods, often without ever connecting the cause with the effect. Your weight-loss saboteurs are typically the foods that you crave and eat at least three times a week. The reactions aren't the same as they are with food allergies, which are immediate reactions to foods (such as hives or the inability to breathe). Instead, these food reactions often cause fatigue, depression, aches, migraines, sinus trouble, and arthritis, among other problems. There are a couple of ways to find out which

THE MOST COMMON FOOD SENSITIVITIES

Food	Frequency of Eating	Do You Crave It?
Sugar		
Wheat (including white-flour products)		
Dairy (milk, cheese, butter, ice cream)		
Corn		
Coffee		
Chocolate		
Eggs		
Beef		
Peanuts		
Soy		
Citrus		
Alcohol		

foods don't like you even though you like them. The first way is educated guessing. Fill out the chart above (you may have to read labels carefully to find hidden foods).

You're probably sensitive to any of the foods listed in the chart that you consume three times a week or more. Any that you crave, you're definitely reactive to, especially the ones you think you can't live without. The reality is that you may not be really living with them. Those favorite foods may make your taste buds feel like they're getting a treat, but it's probably causing that nagging health problem that no one has been able to fix yet.

The Elimination Diet

The best way to find out how things stand is to eliminate all of the foods on the chart that you consume frequently or that you crave. If you suspect you're reactive to certain foods, follow the elimination diet. To properly identify which food or foods may be contributing to your chronic health problems, you'll need to eliminate the suspected foods completely from your diet for a minimum of five days to see whether there's any change. Typically, after noting the improvement, you'll add the foods back into your diet, only one food per day, to see what symptoms (if any) the specific food causes.

You may choose to have an immunoglobulin G (IgG) food-sensitivity blood test that will alert you to which specific foods to avoid and which are probably safe. Another option is to avoid whichever of the following foods you consume daily or a minimum of three times weekly: wheat, dairy, sugar, corn, coffee, chocolate, beef, peanuts, soy, citrus, and alcohol. A third option is to follow the elimination diet, which will effectively eliminate the most commonly reactive foods from your diet as well. Provided that you're having regular daily bowel movements, you'll probably note an improvement in your health by the fifth day of the elimination diet.

During the diet, you should be watching for any changes in your physical health, energy, mood, or mental power. When you add the foods back, a food that causes reactions may cause some unpleasantness. If this occurs, you can use Alka-Seltzer, baking soda, or Thorne's Buffered C Powder (available from your naturopathic physician) in water. This should reduce your adverse reactions within about twenty minutes.

Foods You May Eat
- Cereals. Rice cereals—hot or cold (cream of rice, puffed rice)—and millet.
- Grains. All types of rice except wild rice. Rice pastas are often readily available in the grocery store for you to use. Look for foods labeled Gluten-Free to steer clear of wheat products. Your grocery store or your local health food store should have a good selection of gluten-free products (breads, pastas, cookies).
- Flours. Check the store for gluten-free flours: rice, millet, quinoa, amaranth, teff, bean flours, and buckwheat.
- Meat protein. Lamb, game meats.
- Fish protein. Wild Alaskan salmon, cod, whitefish.
- Soy protein. Tofu, soy cheese.
- Legumes (protein). Beans and nuts (including nut butters)—avoid peanut products and any other nut products that you typically eat three or more times a week.
- Vegetables. Broccoli, green beans, brussels sprouts, cabbage, cauliflower, organic kale, organic celery, organic lettuce, onions,

leeks, parsley, bean sprouts, carrots, sweet potatoes, beets, asparagus, artichokes, squash.

- Oils and fats. Safflower, sunflower, and extra-virgin olive oils.
- Sweeteners. Very small amounts of pure maple syrup, rice bran syrup, and stevia.
- Beverages. Water (plain, mineral, or sparkling), rice or almond milk, teas.
- Condiments. Use salt and pepper and your normal spices as you have been.

Going Gluten-Free

My patients who have come in complaining of allergies have all typically had adverse reactions to wheat as well as sugar. Since gluten intolerance is a common cause of wheat sensitivity, it's often a good idea for people with wheat reactions to go gluten-free. I've been finding gluten intolerance in about 10 percent of my patients, and all have complained of fatigue that went on to improve greatly with elimination of wheat. Wheat can be "hidden" in certain products by being listed as things other than wheat, but it's easy to take all the guesswork out of this diet by simply buying products labeled "gluten-free."

Eliminating wheat and sugar not only gave my patients improved energy and mental functioning, but it also reduced their allergic reactivity. In addition to foods such as cakes, breads, muffins, crackers, cookies, and noodles, look at all labels for the following wheat-containing ingredients:

All-purpose flour
Cake flour
Cereal extract
Durum flour
Enriched flour
Food starch
Gelatin starch
Gluten
Graham flour
Gravies
High-gluten flour
High-protein flour
Hydrolyzed vegetable protein

Malt
Malt extract
Malt flavoring
Modified food starch
Pastry flour
Seitan
Semolina
Semolina flour
Soy sauce
Spelt
Sprouted wheat
Vegetable starch
Wheat bran
Wheat germ

Foods that typically contain wheat include biscuits, breads, cakes, cookies, crackers, crepes, croutons, dumplings, pancakes, pie crusts, pretzels, waffles, noodles, bouillon cubes, soy sauce, processed meats, soups, breaded meats, and breaded vegetables. Don't eat any of these if you're eliminating gluten from your diet.

Foods with Gluten
- Grains, breads, cereals, pastas. Anything made with or containing wheat, barley, rye, oats, spelt, kamut, or triticale; breads and cereals containing wheat starch; cereals and crackers containing wheat or oat bran, graham, wheat germ, or bulgur; cereals and breads containing malt flavoring of unspecified origin; regular spaghetti, macaroni, and noodles; and most packaged rice mixes such as Rice-A-Roni.
- Fruits and vegetables. Products containing thickening agents that may use food starches and stabilizers with gluten (thickening agents often contain wheat flour).
- Meats. Prepared meats, including luncheon meats, sausages, and canned meats containing grain and starch fillers with gluten; fresh ground meats containing Oattrim or LeanMaker; self-basting turkey and other fowl often contain fillers with gluten.

- Dairy products. Cheese foods including spreads, soft cheeses, and dips often contain gluten. Some ice creams may contain gluten stabilizers.
- Salad dressings. Salad dressings containing grain vinegars that include distilled white vinegar (and unspecified vinegars). Some contain emulsifiers and stabilizers with gluten.
- Drinks and juices. Some brands of flavored coffee, herbal tea, and instant cocoa mixes, including malted milk; grain-derived drinks including Postum and Ovaltine.
- Condiments and additives. Products with grain vinegar, including ketchup and mustard; soups and broths containing bouillon; unspecified texturized or hydrolyzed vegetable protein, vegetable gum from oats, and any other product containing an unspecified flour or cereal additive; barley malt; wheat starch; and flavorings made with alcohol. Many soy sauces contain gluten. Caramel candy may contain gluten. Read the labels on margarine packages to check for flour additives. Some spray coatings for nonstick uses have unspecified ingredients added.

Potential Harmful Ingredients
Unidentified starch
Modified food starch
Hydrolyzed vegetable protein—HVP
Hydrolyzed plant protein—HPP
Texturized vegetable protein—TVP
Binders, fillers, excipients, extenders
Malt and other natural flavorings

Gluten may also be used as a binder in some pharmaceutical products. Request clarification from food and drug manufacturers when necessary.

Alcohol and vinegar that are properly distilled should not contain any harmful gluten peptides (or prolomines). Research indicates that the gluten peptide is too large to carry over in the distillation process. This leaves the resultant liquid gluten-free unless a gluten-containing additive is added after the distillation process. Alcohols and vinegars should be carefully investigated for additives before use. Malt vinegars aren't distilled and therefore aren't gluten-free.

Do eat these:

Gluten-Free Foods

- Grains, breads, cereals, pastas. Rice, corn, soy, arrowroot, potato, and tapioca-containing products; breads that contain flour prepared from white or brown rice, potatoes, tapioca, arrowroot, peas, corn, or beans; cereals made from cornmeal, millet, buckwheat, hominy, puffed rice, crisp rice, or cream of rice; malt or malt flavoring derived specifically from corn; pasta made from rice, corn, or beans; and quinoa and amaranth.
- Vegetables. Fresh, frozen, dried, and canned products whose labels indicate that they're free of thickening agents (thickening agents often contain wheat flour).
- Fruits. Fresh, frozen, dried, and canned fruits.
- Meats. Fresh, frozen, and canned meats.
- Dairy products. All aged hard cheeses and pasteurized processed cheeses, including cottage cheese and cream cheese, as well as ice cream that's free of gluten stabilizers. Most children with celiac disease tolerate milk and yogurt containing milk sugar (lactose) soon after starting a gluten-free diet.
- Salad dressings. Many but not all salad dressings are gluten-free. Apple, wine, and rice vinegars are generally acceptable.
- Condiments and additives. Soy sauce that doesn't contain wheat or barley hydrolyzed or textured soy and corn vegetable protein; corn malt; starch (raw or modified from arrowroot, corn, potatoes, and tapioca); and vegetable gum from carob, locust bean, cellulose gum, guar gum, gum arabic, gum acacia, gum tragacanth, or xanthan gum.
- Drinks and juices. Freshly brewed coffee, tea, chocolate made from powdered cocoa, carbonated drinks, and juices made from fresh fruit.

  Wine, rum, tequila, and sake are usually safe, as their alcohols don't generally come from toxic grains. Some vodkas are also okay. However, as with any ingested product, you should gauge your reaction and learn as much about your favored brands as possible.

Alcohol appears to have the ability to concentrate and carry the allergic portion of all of the foods that were used to make it. So it's often highly reactive for people with allergies to grain (including gluten), sugar, and yeast.

Many kinds of liquor are made with grain alcohol and so may be suspect. Whiskey, bourbon, gin, and rye are definitely off the list, since they're made with rye and barley. Beer, too, must be avoided, since malt (usually from barley) is an ingredient. Even rice beers use malt.

Avoiding Dairy

Besides sugar and wheat, dairy is the other most common reactive food, and if you don't see enough improvement after cutting out sugar and wheat, try quitting dairy, too. Dairy is typically pretty easy to identify, as it includes anything with milk, cream, ice cream, cheese, cream cheese, cottage cheese, sour cream, or yogurt. It can also be listed on the ingredient list as one of the following:

Casein
Casein hydrolysates
Curds
Ghee
Lactalbumin
Lactoglobulin
Lactose
Lactulose
Milk solids
Rennet
Whey
Whey hydrolysates

Milk is usually found in the following products:
• Baking powder biscuits, breads, pancakes, waffles, flour mixes
• Doughnuts, cakes, cookies, pie crusts, puddings, muffins, popovers, caramel, curds, custards

- Omelets and scrambled eggs if cheese is added
- Chocolate (milk or dark), cocoa drinks, Ovaltine, malted milk, milkshakes, ice cream
- Milk-based salad dressings; creamed foods, soups, and casseroles; chowders; cream sauces; scalloped dishes; Alfredo sauce
- Fritters, buttered popcorn, gravies, mashed potatoes, battered foods

If you want more confirmation before jumping into this diet, go to your local naturopathic physician or holistic doctor and get a blood test for food reactions. This test will measure an immune marker, typically IgG, in your blood against a number of foods. It will probably turn out that you're reactive to the foods that you have a lot of antibodies against. I recommend that any foods with IgG levels reaching even the low range be taken out of the diet for two weeks and then added back in as I mentioned previously. (The resource section includes lists of foods that commonly contain wheat, dairy, and gluten.)

Go Green

At this point you may be thinking, "That's everything I eat! What can I eat?" This is a common response, as we typically eat various combinations of those sugar, wheat, and dairy products on a regular basis. For some people, that's virtually all they eat. So finding alternatives can take some time. Start with the food you love and consume the most. Identify where it is in your diet and look for alternatives. Check your local health food stores as well as the local grocery store and experiment with what they have to offer. When you find a replacement that works for you—and tastes good—make the switch.

1. Eat a Rainbow of Colors

If your diet isn't colorful, now is the time to make it rich in greens, reds, oranges, purples, and yellows. The greens are especially important, and you should be working on ways to eat them every day—lots of them. Remember, the green color is from chlorophyll, which will escort toxic chemicals out of your body. So make greens your friends.

Vegetables

Eat at least five and up to nine servings of vegetables every day. A serving is about half a cup. They can be fresh or frozen, but don't use canned. Use the darkest-colored vegetables you can. It's best to steam them or quickly stir-fry them in a wok. Limit how long you cook them to keep most of the goodness inside the vegetables.

Be sure you eat at least one of the Brassicas every day: broccoli, cauliflower, cabbage, brussels sprouts, and kale. Also include some of the yellow, orange, and red veggies (sweet potatoes, carrots, and tomatoes).

For salads, use leaf lettuce or organic salad mixes, which are readily available at most stores. Try adding some dried fruit, nuts, and cheeses to the salad. Experiment with olive oil and a high-quality balsamic vinegar. Avoid fat-free dressings, as they prevent you from absorbing the beneficial carotene compounds from the vegetables in the salad.

Avoid buying or eating commercial varieties of any of the twelve most toxic fruits and vegetables: peaches, apples, sweet bell peppers, celery, nectarines, strawberries, cherries, pears, imported grapes, spinach, lettuce, and potatoes.

Fruit

Eat one or two pieces of fruit a day. Morning seems to be the best time to eat fruit, before our digestion gets going. But you can also snack on fruit. Try cutting up an organic apple and putting some organic nut butter on the slices.

2. Eat More Vegetarian Protein Sources

We've already covered the fact that a diet with a good amount of lean protein is very helpful in clearing chemical toxins more rapidly from the bloodstream, but having vegetable-based protein in the diet is even better. All of the published studies on healthy diets continue to prove that the more vegetarian one's diet is, the healthier one is. So dig into the following:

- Beans, peas, lentils. Be sure to soak the beans overnight and add an inch or two of the seaweed kombu (available at most health food stores) to help reduce the gas. Discard the water they were soaked in and use new water to cook. Lentils don't require soaking. There are many wonderful and flavorful beans available that can be mixed together for soups and other bean dishes. Canned organic beans are also available. To reduce the time it takes to make beans for dinner, you can either start them in the slow cooker in the morning before you leave for work or cook them in a pressure cooker when you get home.

- Nuts. Raw nuts are best, except for peanuts, which should be eaten only after roasting or boiling. Be sure the nuts haven't gone rancid. If they leave a bad taste in your mouth, the oils in the nuts have gone rancid—don't eat them.
- Nut butters. Many wonderful nut butters are available. It's best to buy organic to avoid the partially hydrogenated oils that nonorganic varieties add. Look for other butters besides just peanut—try almond and cashew butters.
- Soy products. Soy is a very healthy food and is thought to be protective against breast and prostate cancers.
- Tofu. This is one of the most common soy foods and is very easy to work with. For ideas on how to use it, just search for tofu recipes on the Internet. You can bake it with some type of salad dressing or sauce and then add it to your stir-fries, soups, or other dishes. It can also be scrambled in the morning with vegetables (if you add cumin seasoning, it will turn yellow just like eggs).
- Soy meats. Various soy burgers and soy sausages are available.
- Soy dairy alternatives. Soy milk and cheeses are available for those who are reactive to dairy but not to soy.

If you eat meat, dairy, or fish, make sure it's clean and green.

Meat

The best meats to eat on a regular basis are game meats or organically raised meats. A number of Internet sources for organic meats are available, and there may well be a meat market in your area that specializes in game meats. Here are some of them:

www.maverickranch.com
www.grasslandbeef.com
www.pratherranch.com

Many people with severe food reactions to meats have found relief when rotating the different game meats and using organic sources.

Keep in mind that all of the studies have shown that people who eat the least amount of meats are the healthiest and typically the thinnest. Don't eat meats more than once a day. If you're blood type A, you should probably be eating meats only occasionally because you probably don't have the ability to fully digest meat.

Avoid processed meats. Hot dogs (anyone who has ever visited a hot dog manufacturing company will never eat a hot dog again), salami, pepperoni, bacon, and so forth. These are poor-quality meats and are often full of nitrates and other preservatives that will not preserve your health. Please avoid them.

Fish

Eat oily fish two or three times weekly. The best fish to eat is wild Alaskan salmon (either king, red, or silver). It's available fresh at stores and restaurants only from June through September. It's available at some stores in the frozen section and as canned salmon throughout the year. You can also get excellent Alaskan salmon from www.vitalchoice.com.

Do not eat farmed or Atlantic salmon, which is the most commonly available form of salmon. This is a highly contaminated (toxic) food. Avoid tuna, orange roughy, swordfish, shark, halibut, and snapper, as these all have high levels of mercury. Cod, whitefish, and tilapia are great alternatives.

Here's a list of the most commonly available low-mercury fish:

Clams
Ocean perch
Alaskan salmon
Shrimp
Tilapia
Flounder or sole
Scallops
Catfish

Eggs

Use organic eggs. Eggs are the gold standard for a complete protein.

Dairy

It's best to buy organic varieties, since nonorganic versions can contain fat-soluble toxins.

- Butter. Always buy organic.
- Milk. Use the lowest-fat version that agrees with your taste buds.
- Cheese. Use low-fat cheeses.
- Yogurt. Always use plain and then add your own fruit. The pre-mixed yogurts are way too high in sugar and high-fructose corn syrup, which is very unhealthy.

Eat Good Fat

It's very important to get healthy oils in our diets. The healthy oils are often called essential because it's essential that we include them in our diet. These are mostly liquid at room temperature, while the not-so-healthy fats and oils are typically solid at room temperature.

Look for good oils: butter (organic), extra-virgin olive oil, and safflower and sunflower seed oils. Most oils need to be refrigerated, but olive oil can just be stored in a cool, dark cabinet. It's best to buy olive oil in dark bottles.

Eat Whole Grains—but Not Too Much

Always use whole grains. Find the whole-grain breads, mixes, and pastas to use instead of those with refined flours.

- Crackers. Buy whole-grain crackers without partially hydrogenated oils in them. If you're avoiding wheat, look for rice crackers, rice cakes, RyKrisp, Wasa, Ak-Mak, and other whole-grain crackers.
- Hot cereals. Avoid the prepackaged, just-add-water cereals. These are often loaded with sugars and other things you don't need. Use the whole-grain cereals—make real oatmeal, grits, or cream of rice. Making hot cereal from whole grains or some of these packaged products (such as grits, cream of rice) takes only a short time. When making rolled oats, add some dried fruits and nuts to the water. Cinnamon is great, too.

- Cold cereals. Lots of healthy low-sugar cold cereals are available, including wheat- and gluten-free cereals. If you can't find them at your local grocery store, check your health food store.

3. Find Delicious Replacements

This may be one of the most fun parts of this plan. Take a slow, leisurely tour of the health food aisle at your local grocery store and make an excursion to the two nearest organic stores, too. With your list of favorites in hand, peruse the aisles and look for better alternatives. Keep trying different brands and varieties until you find a few you love.

In addition to finding healthy replacements for your favorite foods, you can start trying the recipes that Kelly and I have provided in chapter 8 after week four of the plan. We've shared recipes for breakfasts, lunches, and dinners that are healthy, delicious, and relatively easy to make.

Although many of the recipes will take only about thirty minutes to prepare, you may want to devote some time to making them on the weekend so they're readily available during the week. (You may also want to check with your local health food store for cooking classes.) Getting the hang of your new way of eating will probably take a couple of weeks, but you will undoubtedly start to feel better by the end of the first week!

Week 2: Your Home on a Diet

Continue practicing the guidelines from week one while you begin following this week's guidelines.

Your Goal: To remove the toxins from your home and replace them with green alternatives.

You'll begin by getting rid of the most toxic products in your home, such as pesticides and scented dryer sheets, and then assess the bigger improvements you'd like to make, like replacing particleboard furniture pieces or getting rid of the carpeting and putting in wood or tile flooring. You'll also be checking for hidden mold and figuring out how to keep the air that circulates through your home as clean as possible.

Get Clean

It's time to fill that trash can!

1. Find and Evict the Hidden Enemies

The first step is not to bring any more chemical compounds into your home that will contaminate the air. Transforming your home to be as least toxic as possible can take some time to fully realize. But with the simple steps that follow, you can accomplish a lot with very little effort.

Breathe cleaner air by evicting:

Aromatic hydrocarbons from combustion
Chloroforms
Heavy metals
Mold toxins
Pesticides
Plastics
Solvents

Dispose of cosmetics and personal hygiene products that contain:

Chlorinated pesticides
Heavy metals
PCBs
Solvents

Make your home a shoe-free zone by making it easy to remove and store your shoes at the front door. At our house, we provide warm, comfy slippers for family and friends.

Definitely make your home smoke free. As you learned in chapter 6, smoking produces some of the worst indoor air pollutants.

If you have your clothes dry-cleaned, let them air out in the garage before bringing them into the house. Better yet, have your clothes wet-cleaned, a new process that incorporates biodegradable soaps and works just as well.

YOUR CLEANING CHECKLIST

Home Exposure	Yes	No	If the Answer Is Yes	Done
Do you use pesticide sprays for the home or garden?			Stop using them and safely discard the cans.	
Do you have scented candles in the house?			Take them out of the house.	
Do you have metal-wicked candles (slow-burning) in the house?			Take them out of the house.	
Do you use air fresheners in the house?			Don't use air fresheners; instead remove sources of objectionable odors.	
Do you have plug-in air fresheners in the house?			Take them out of the house.	
Do you use scented dryer sheets?			Switch to unscented dryer sheets.	
Do you use scented laundry detergent?			Switch to unscented detergent.	
Do you use aerosol sprays in the house?			Switch to nonaerosol sprays (such as pump-action sprays).	
Do you cook with Teflon pans?			Switch to pans without Teflon.	
Do you cook with aluminum pans?			Switch to nonaluminum pans.	
Do you have powerful household spray cleaners for use in your home?			Replace with vinegar, baking soda, or other safe cleaners.	
Do you use a soap-scum cleaner for your shower?			Begin to use a squeegee to clean the walls after each shower.	
Do you wear perfumes or colognes?			Look for natural fragrances that do not have solvents and other chemicals.	

At this point, you've done a tremendous amount to reduce the load of toxic chemicals in the air. As you must have noticed, the majority of these changes were very simple and easy to accomplish.

2. Deep Cleaning

Mold is one of the most insidious hidden enemies and can cause an array of health problems, including asthma, allergies, decreased ability to think and remember things, and immune problems. I'm currently working with someone who reacted to mold by retaining water and bloating. She said it looked as if she were three months pregnant—and she was right.

MOLD CHECK

Home Exposure	Yes	No	If the Answer Is Yes
Has there been water damage in your house?			Immediately call a professional and have your home checked for mold. Then have the mold remediated by professionals.
Is there anywhere in your home that smells musty or moldy?			Same as above: act immediately.
Can you see mold somewhere in your home?			Same as above: act immediately.

A lot of the toxins that you breathe at home are being circulated by your furnace and central air-conditioning through the air ducts.

AIR CHECK

Cleaning Maintenance	Yes	No	If the Answer Is Yes
Has it been more than a year since your air ducts have been cleaned out?			Get a professional service to come in and clean the ducts. But don't let them spray chemicals into the ducts afterward.
Has it been longer than three months since you've changed your furnace filters (or longer than one month if you have pets)?			Replace your filters with pleated filters rated MERV 7–9.

Go Green

Here's what you need to add to your home to make it healthier.

1. Breathe Easy

The changes you're making are going a long way toward making your home a toxin-free zone, and if you're not already feeling a little better, expect it to happen within days. Meanwhile, you can consider the following suggestions for making your air even greener.

For starters, invest in a high-quality air filter for your home. (The best are listed in the resource section.) This is particularly important if you have electronic and office equipment in your home that will off-gas plastic fumes and ozone.

It's also important to use an air filter because many of the materials used to build homes off-gas chemicals that could be negatively affecting your health. Your new air filter should clear the air in your home (or bedroom) at least once every thirty minutes. (See chapter 6

HOME IMPROVEMENT CHECK

Home Exposure	Yes	No	If the Answer Is Yes
Is your water supply treated with chlorine?			Install chlorine filters on your showers (available at all hardware/home supply stores)
Are you planning on painting the inside of your home?			Check with your local Environmental Building Center (or look on the Web) for chemically safe paints. (Low-VOC paints can have lots of other toxic compounds in them.)
Do you have gas appliances?			Consider replacing them with electric. Meanwhile, have the gas utility check for gas leaks and CO levels.
Do you have particleboard furniture in your home?			Remove it. Then begin looking for replacements made with real wood.
Do you have wall-to-wall carpeting?			Remove it. Consider replacing it with prefinished real wood flooring, tile, or stone. (Note: stone and tile floors can have electric heating elements placed below them so that your feet stay warm.)

for instructions on how to compute cubic feet per minute.) If you have a home ionizer or ozone generator, stop using it and replace it with a high-quality air purifier.

You also want to keep dirty air from recirculating. Ironically, the biggest offender is probably your most-used cleaning machine—the vacuum. Unless it's equipped with a HEPA filter, a lot of dust is being blown right back into your air.

2. Make Green Improvements

Now we're getting down to the changes that will often take more time, planning, and finances and may require the services of some professionals as well.

Week 3: Out with the Bad

Keep working on what you started in weeks one and two. Sometimes it takes a while to find good replacements for foods you're used to eating and products you're used to using, so don't worry if this takes more than a week. The most important thing is that you're clearly on your way. Completing weeks one and two—eliminating toxin exposures via your food and your home air—will allow you to move on to this week's mission: cleansing.

Your Goal: To get all of your body's elimination systems operating at full efficiency.

Get Clean

I tell my patients that it's best to plug the hole in the boat before you start bailing. In other words, prevent more water from getting aboard before focusing on dumping what's already there. Otherwise, you're simply keeping up at best, rather than getting ahead and fixing the problem. And now that you've done that—now that you've taken measures to prevent toxins from getting "aboard"—let's start bailing some of your internal toxic load.

1. Clean Your Primary Exit Route

Start with making sure your exit routes are in proper working order before moving lots of toxins through them. The primary route to be concerned with is your bowels. It's ideal if you're having two or three well-formed bowel movements a day, but if you're constipated, your first goal is to have a daily movement. The first step in any cleansing program is to make sure you're having regular bowel movements. If you're constipated, you're completely unable to clear out any fat-soluble toxins. This obviously leads to an increased toxic load in your body, making you feel even lousier than the constipation itself can be blamed for.

There are several reasons for constipation:

- For many people, consuming sugar and the most common reactive foods can cause it. So, having made the changes in week one may already be improving your regularity. If you haven't yet been successful at eliminating these foods, please give it another try.
- Some people become constipated if they aren't producing enough hydrochloric acid (HCL) in their stomachs to properly digest all of their food. When that happens, food tends to sit in the stomach like a brick, taking an eternity to digest. Gas buildup can also result; it's common in people who have type A blood. If you think this is what is happening with you, you may want to see a naturopathic physician before trying supplementation with HCL during your meals.

If you have constipation that's characterized by hard, dry stools:

- Drink more water, which in itself is necessary for cleansing.
- Take magnesium every day (at least 500 milligrams). Magnesium is one of the most commonly deficient nutrients in chemically burdened people, and when that's the case, the body will pull all of the magnesium out of the intestines to share the supply. While this is good for the rest of the body, it's bad for the bowels, since magnesium holds water in the stool, making it moist and easy to pass. It works best to take the low-cost magnesium tablets from your local pharmacy or grocery store. These aren't absorbed well, so they stay in your intestines and will make your stools moister and easier to pass within just a few days.

To make your digestive system stronger, begin taking a probiotic product (healthy bacteria for your intestines), such as HMF (available from your naturopathic physician) or Kyo-Dophilus (available at most health food stores). Typically, one cap a day is sufficient.

Once your bowels are open, you can begin to increase the amount of toxins passing through them. This can be accomplished simply by adding certain foods and supplements to your diet, but you'll get much faster results by starting a regimen of colonic irrigations.

Colon Hydrotherapy

In my practice, this has been the toughest thing to get patients to do (next to getting them to stop eating the favorite foods that they're reacting adversely to), but the benefits are enormous. In my office, we've documented chlorinated pesticides and heavy metals leaving the body during colonics. Wouldn't it be nice to document toxins leaving your body, too?

Effects
- Allows the liver to dump toxic bile and have those toxins escorted out of the body.
- Increases the movement of heavy metals out of the bowels.
- Normalizes peristalsis and elimination.
- Helps restore proper bowel function when one has regular constipation or diarrhea.

Indications
- Constipation or diarrhea
- Atonic, or "lazy," bowels
- Poor digestion—bloating, gas
- Hemorrhoids
- Toxic conditions—chronic headaches, skin disorders, allergies, asthma, eczema, detoxification of liver, autoimmune conditions, fibromyalgia, fatigue
- Halitosis
- Candida

Contraindications
- Colon cancer, polyps, or colon surgery
- Pregnancy

- Appendicitis
- Abdominal pain of unknown origin
- Acute inflammation—acute ulcerative colitis, acute Crohn's disease, fissures and inflamed hemorrhoids, diverticulitis
- Rectal bleeding
- Congestive heart failure, hypertension

Check with your naturopathic physician, chiropractor, or health food store owner to get information on who in your area does a great job. If no one fits the description, try getting your own machine (see resource section).

How Often Should You Get a Colonic?

Consider doing colonic irrigations on a regular basis to dramatically reduce your toxic burden in a shorter length of time. To see whether this is going to help, schedule them twice a week for two weeks. One colonic a week seems to keep the toxic load from building, but two or more a week will lower the burden and allow you to see the difference it makes. Then, to keep feeling good after those first two weeks, you'll need to continue with the colonics once or twice a week. Most of my cleansing patients end up doing them at least twice a week for a few months before they slow down on them. Your body will guide you in this process.

To increase the amount of toxic compounds that are getting out with each colonic, you can get Liver Cleanse (Thorne Research) from your naturopathic physician (it isn't sold through health food stores) and begin taking one or two the night before your colonic irrigation. While doing colonics, take probiotic supplements and consume drinks that replace electrolytes, such as a good vegetable juice or Emergen-C drink powder mixed with water.

You don't need to be concerned about the safety of colonics as long as they're done with a certified colon therapist on a good machine. A recent study done in Great Britain revealed that none of the participants, some of whom did hundreds of colonics, had experienced any adverse effects. Home units are an option for those who have done colonics with therapists and know how their bodies respond to the process. See the resource section for information about these units.

2. Optimize Your Kidney and Liver Function

We also want to ensure that you aren't recycling a lot of toxins in your kidneys and that your liver is clean enough to effectively handle the toxins you're dumping. Alkalinize your urine by following the dietary changes in chapter 3, using a multiple vitamin with citrate forms of the minerals, and drinking glass-bottled sparkling water and stinging nettle tea.

Use Old-Fashioned Castor Oil Packs to Detox Your Liver

You will need the following materials to make your own castor oil pack:

- Castor oil. You can find this at the local drugstore or health food store. The best castor oil to use for a pack is from Heritage, which should be available at the health food store.
- An old towel you don't care about that's large enough to cover your abdomen.
- A heating pad.

Directions for use:

1. Typically, the castor oil pack is laid over the liver for people undergoing any cleansing protocols. But it can also be laid over any area of your body that's in pain (as long as there's no wound in that area).
2. For the liver, apply a generous portion of castor oil over your liver area and cover completely with the towel.
3. Put the heating pad over the towel (so that the castor oil does not soak into the heating pad) and turn it on.
4. Keep the castor oil pack in place for thirty minutes. Do not fall asleep and leave the heating pad on all night.
5. After removing the pad, you can clean the area with soap or baking soda in water.
6. The towel will never be free of the castor oil, so keep that in mind when laundering.

Healing Foods for the Liver

Historically, apples have been thought to stimulate all body secretions. They contain malic acid and tartaric acid, which help prevent liver troubles. Cherries and dandelion greens are very cleansing to the liver. And dandelion tea has been used for centuries to help the liver, as has turmeric. Grapefruit, parsley, pomegranate, quince, raspberries, strawberries, tangerines, and tomatoes are thought to help relieve a sluggish liver and liver congestion. Watercress relieves inflammation of the liver, and garlic can be helpful as well. Eating artichokes, beets, radishes, and any of the brassicas (broccoli, cauliflower, cabbage, kale, brussels sprouts) is also very helpful. Avoid all alcohol, sugar, and high-fat meals as well. Here's the complete list of foods good for the liver:

Apple juice (organic)
Apples (organic)
Artichokes
Beet greens
Beet juice
Beets
Broccoli
Brussels sprouts
Cauliflower
Cranberries
Curcumin (turmeric)
Dandelions (tea, wine, leaves)
Endive
Garlic
Gooseberries
Grape juice
Grapefruit
Grapes (U.S. or organic)
Green peppers (organic)
Green tea
Kale
Milk thistle
Olives
Pomegranates
Quinces
Radishes

Raspberries
Rooibos
Rosemary (organic)
Spinach (organic)
Strawberries
Tangerines
Turnip greens
Watercress
White tea

3. Detox Through Your Skin

While the bowels, kidneys, and liver do the lion's share of elimination, the skin is the body's largest organ and shouldn't be ignored.

Brush Your Skin

Dry skin brushing is very helpful before and after a sauna and before the colonic irrigations. Dry skin brushing is a time-honored method of increasing the movement of lymph in the body. Lymph is a serum that bathes the blood cells, picks up waste material, then moves through lymphatic tissue, and eventually dumps back into the bloodstream. The lymphatic system has been described as the body's garbage-collecting system. The system doesn't have a heart to pump the lymph through the lymph channels, as happens with the blood, so to move the lymph through the body, you need to exercise, get a massage, or do dry skin brushing. Brushing with a good natural bristle brush helps move lymph that's close to the surface of the skin.

Brush from the ends of your arms and legs toward the core of your body, and then move from there toward the heart. The brushes are available at most health food stores.

Take a Low-Temperature Sauna

Sauna therapy is another valuable tool for mobilizing fat-soluble toxins from fat stores. Toxins residing in the pads of fat just under the skin can be moved through the skin and out of the body by the sweat produced. Toxins stored in the fat pads deeper inside the body will be mobilized into the bloodstream, just as would happen with weight loss. Sauna therapy is for people who have high levels of circulating toxins and should be done only after they've started colonics or some other means to enhance the body's ability to force toxins to leave through the bowels. Otherwise, their bloodstreams will be flooded with toxins that may then cause more damage. Saunas can be done once a week, and it's best to do them before the colonic, not after. Follow these tips when taking a sauna:

- Keep the sauna at about 135 degrees Fahrenheit, and work your way up from a thirty-minute stay to a sixty-minute stay.
- Be sure to take electrolyte replacements after the sauna and drink lots of water.
- Be sure that the sauna isn't made of plastic or plywood and doesn't contain a lot of glues, as these would all be off-gassing in the sauna while you're in there.

Go Green

Now that your bowels and kidneys are working better and you aren't recycling as many toxins, you can begin to increase the movement of these toxins out through those exit routes. The easiest way to approach this is with the foods that you put into your mouth.

1. Eat More Whole-Grain Brown Rice, Greens, and Special Agents

Increase the amount of whole-grain brown rice and green vegetables in your diet. The recipes that appear in chapter 8 will help you achieve that.

- Eat brown rice on a daily basis. If you can't, take three capsules of a rice bran fiber supplement with each meal to enhance the excretion of fat-soluble toxins. If the rice bran fiber is in powder form, take one scoop with each meal.
- Eat dark green vegetables daily, at every meal, if possible.
- If you don't yet like to eat green vegetables every day, take a daily supplement that includes green food extracts or enjoy one of the many green drinks available, such as Daily Greens or Liquid Life (with broccoli extract). You can drink an ounce of liquid extracts, a green juice, or use one of the green powders.

- Eat foods that reduce the recycling of toxins by increasing your dietary intake of organic varieties of:
  Apples
  Beans
  Blackberries
  Cherries
  Lentils
  Melons
  Pears
  Plums
  Soy
  Squash
  Strawberries
  Zucchini

2. Get Your Daily Quota of Green Tea and Herbs

Drinking green tea daily has been shown to enhance excretion of fat-soluble toxins. It has many other health benefits as well, including cancer-fighting properties and the power to enhance and preserve brain function.

It's best to drink 20 ounces of green tea three times a day. The longer you leave the tea bags in the cup, the more power you get. For those who don't want to actually drink green tea, many green tea extracts are available as liquids and capsules. Typically, one capsule is all you would need (most capsules contain the polyphenols found in two or three cups of tea). You can also begin consuming saponin-containing herbs to inhibit your pancreatic lipase, which will increase the amount of fat in your stools that escorts toxins out of your body (see resource section). These herbs include:

Horse chestnut (available at most health food stores)—2 capsules daily

Panax ginseng (available at all health food stores)—2 capsules daily

Gotu kola (available at many health food stores)—2 capsules daily

Now that you've completed week three, you've dramatically reduced the amount of toxins that are being recycled back into your bloodstream and have increased the amount of toxins exiting your body. With just these first two clean and green steps, you've started to reverse the buildup of toxins in your body that's been going on since you were born. Even if you did nothing else to boost the amount of toxins leaving your body, over time you would be able to achieve a great many of your health goals.

Week 4: Put the Toxin-Fighting Supplements to Work

Now that you're taking in fewer toxins and more efficiently getting rid of the ones you have, it's time to start taking some supplements that will move the toxins out of your body faster and build your strength, energy, and overall health.

Your Goal: To accelerate the reduction of your toxic load and increase your overall health by taking supplements.

The following lists contain the basic supplements that we all need to help us handle the toxic environment we're currently living in, along with necessary supplements for anyone doing any form of cleansing and those aimed at speeding up fat loss. As I've mentioned, I take a lot more supplements than that, simply because I know too much about the environment, our diet, and health not to.

Get Clean

These are the supplements that I think are the absolute minimum that everyone should be taking just to stay on an even keel in our environment. These are the nutrients that we are deficient in because of our daily toxin exposures (and the toxic burden that we carry), and the nutrients that will help us metabolize the toxins and keep them from doing much damage.

The dosages I recommend exceed the official recommended daily allowances, and there's a good reason for that—the severity of our toxic burden calls for more serious measures.

UNITED STATES RECOMMENDED DIETARY ALLOWANCES (RDA)

Compound	Units	Adult Males	Adult Females	Children 7 to 10 Years	Infants	Pregnant and Lactating Women*
Protein	g	63	50	28	14	65
Vitamin A	RE*	1000	800	700	375	1300
Vitamin D	IU	200	200	400	400	400
Vitamin E	mg alphaTE*	10	8	7	4	12
Vitamin K	mg	80	65	30	10	65
Vitamin C	mg	60	60	45	35	95
Folate	µg	200	180	100	35	400
Thiamine (B1)	mg	1.5	1.1	1	0.4	1.6
Riboflavin (B2)	mg	1.7	1.3	1.2	0.5	1.8
Niacin	mg	19	15	13	6	20
Pyridoxine (B6)	mg	2	1.6	1.4	0.6	2.2
Cyanocobalamine (B12)	µg	2	2	1,4	0.5	2.6
Biotin	mg	30–100	30–100	30	15	30–100
Pantothenic acid	mg	4–7	4–7	4–5	3	4–7
Calcium (Ca)	mg	800	800	800	600	1200
Phosphorus (P)	mg	800	800	800	500	1200
Iodine (I)	µg	150	150	120	50	200
Iron (Fe)	mg	10	15	10	10	30
Magnesium (Mg)	mg	350	280	170	60	355
Copper (Cu)	mg	1.5–3	1.5–3	1–2	0.6–0.7	1.5–3
Zinc (Zn)	mg	15	12	10	5	19
Selenium (Se)	µg	70	55	30	15	75
Chromium (Cr)	µg	50–200	50–200	50–200	10–60	50–200
Molybdenum (Mo)	µg	75–250	75–250	50–150	15–40	75–250
Manganese (Mn)	mg	2–5	2–5	2–3	0.3–1.0	2–5
Fluoride (F)	mg	1.5–4	1.5–4	1.5–2.5	0.1–1	1.5–4
Sodium (Na)	mg	500	500	400	120–200	500
Chloride (Cl)	mg	750	750	600	180–300	750
Potassium (K)	mg	2000	2000	1600	500–700	2000

Source: Recommended Daily Allowances: National Academy of Sciences; 10th ed., 1989.
g = grams; mg = milligrams (0.001 g); µg = micrograms (0.000001 g); IU = International Units; RE = Retinol Equivalent; AlphaTE = alpha Tocopherol equivalent.

*Generally the higher number was reported.

1. Take a Multiple Vitamin and Mineral Daily

Your multivitamins should have a combination of all of the normal vitamins and minerals, with a little more of each of the following common ingredients:

Vitamin B1 — 100 mg
Vitamin B2 — 50 mg
Vitamin B6 — 100 mg
Magnesium — 500 mg
Alpha-lipoic acid — 50 mg
N-acetyl-L-cysteine (NAC) — 100 mg
Selenium — 200 mcg

In addition to higher levels of these nutrients, the best multivitamins for dealing with toxicity also contain extracts of:

Broccoli
Dandelion (*Taraxacum*)
Green tea
Milk thistle
Turmeric (curcumin)
Rooibos

If you can't find any locally, check the resource section.

2. Supplement Your Multivitamin

You should supplement your multivitamin or mineral with the cleaning powers of the following:

- Vitamin C. Begin with 3,000 milligrams a day. If you're a smoker or live with one, you'll need to double this amount. That also goes for those who drive a lot or live in highly polluted urban areas. I typically have my most toxic patients on a total of at least 9,000 milligrams. Some people will experience diarrhea if they go above 1,000 milligrams a day; if you're one of them, just don't take any more than that.

- Magnesium. Start with one capsule of about 150 milligrams a day and build up to three or more doses a day. You'll know you've had enough when you start having loose stools. Just notch it back by a dose at that point. Because magnesium is one of the most commonly deficient nutrients in people with chemical overload, it's important to take as much as your body can comfortably tolerate.
- Good fiber to help usher the toxins out of the body. The best is one that's mostly rice bran fiber, with some psyllium added. Many fiber products are mostly or solely psyllium. While psyllium is a great fiber, I've found that about 30 percent of my patients are reactive to it and will become constipated (the exact opposite of what I'm aiming for). Begin with one scoop or three to four capsules of rice bran fiber after each meal.
- High-quality whey protein powder. Add two scoops a day to juice or soy milk (if you aren't reactive to soy). This will help to make more glutathione and will help your liver to clear toxins from the bloodstream. The higher the quality of the whey, the more glutathione it will make and the more it will cost—but it's worth it. See the resource section for high-quality whey.

Go Green

In addition to taking supplements that help you with cleansing, you want to be sure you're getting what your body needs to build and repair any damage done by the toxins. As I've mentioned, I take a lot more supplements than those listed above.

1. Supplements for Cleansing and Weight-Loss

Take the supplements I've found to be a necessary part of any cleansing and weight-loss program. They include:

- Chlorophyll. If you aren't eating a lot of green veggies, take one ounce of a liquid extract, one bottle of a green drink, or a scoop of greens powder.
- Probiotics. Take one capsule a day. Probiotics such as acidophilus provide good bacteria that the intestines need to stay healthy. A recent study of more than 900 chemically toxic Americans

revealed that probiotics were the supplement they found most helpful. There's also evidence in the scientific literature that these healthy bacteria prevent the absorption of some toxins from the gastrointestinal tract.

- *N*-acetyl-L-cysteine. Take 1,500 milligrams a day. This nutrient helps increase the amount of glutathione in the body, a main defender against environmental toxins. This is especially important if you live in an area with high pollution. I make sure I take more on the days when I go out riding my bike, even though much of my ride is through the Arizona desert, which isn't highly polluted.

- Vitamin E. Take an extra 400 to 500 units above the amount in your multivitamins. Vitamin E is a potent antioxidant that can cross your blood-brain barrier and protect those brain cells from damage from pesticides and other chemicals. It has also been very effective over the years at helping to protect arteries from hardening and preventing plaque from building up.

- Fish oils. Have at least 1,500 milligrams daily of these essential oils, which are very helpful in maintaining good health. The DHA portion of fish oil is one of the best ways to protect the brain from damage from the ever-present organophosphate pesticides. If you have a lot of inflammation in your body, you can increase the dose to 3,000 milligrams daily.

- Liquid Life, a liquid extract with 250 milligrams of blackberry, elderberry, wolfberry, mangosteen, broccoli, and green tea extracts per ounce. Have 1 ounce a day. This is a very potent product that helps restore, preserve, and optimize mitochondrial function; protect the heart; and optimize the immune, cardiovascular, and blood sugar systems.

- Ginkgo biloba. Take one capsule of a ginkgo solid extract daily for mitochondrial protection, and the extra protection for the brain and the other functional brain benefits.

2. Accelerate Your Weight Loss

Even with the bases well covered by the nutrients listed previously, some of you may still want some additional focused help to speed up fat loss. Since your liver and exit routes are now well equipped to handle an increased movement of fat from your storehouses (and the chemicals that will move into the blood with the fat), you can begin to work with the following compounds:

- Green tea (yes, I'm listing it here again—it has so many fantastic benefits!)—2 cups of strong green tea (not the decaf kind) to help with weight loss as well as clearing compounds from the body.
- Cayenne—use this to spice up your meals on a daily basis. You don't need much. Or use 0.4 to 1.0 milligram of capsaicin extract a day—a little goes a long way.
- Conjugated linoleic acid—3,000–4,000 milligrams a day for an added weight-loss boost.

Finally, here are some herbs and spices that you shouldn't mind supplementing your diet with in the name of heading off or easing aches, pains, and other inconveniences.

- Basil. This herb is rich in antioxidants and it's an antimicrobial, so it blocks the progress of viruses that cause colds. Take 1 to 2 tablespoons a day.
- Cinnamon. This spice contains a polyphenol compound that enhances insulin's function, reducing blood sugar levels and therefore fighting diabetes. Take ½ teaspoon a day.
- Garlic. In studies conducted at the Linus Pauling Institute, people who took this antioxidant herb from the lily family for three months experienced a total cholesterol reduction of 6 percent to 11 percent. Eat three to five crushed cloves a day.
- Nutmeg. Warming spices such as nutmeg lower blood pressure by drawing blood from the body's center toward the skin (hence the warming), dispersing the blood, and lowering the pressure. Eat ½ to 1 teaspoon a day.
- Clove. This spice contains a phytochemical that bars the path of a protein complex associated with arthritis. Take ½ teaspoon a day.
- Thyme. This antispasmodic herb can ease coughing, and its antiseptic properties combat inflammation of the throat. Take 2 to 3 teaspoons a day.

You Did It!

Gather your team members and have a nice cup of green tea together with some gluten-free muffins. You've just succeeded in making a huge life change, an "I love myself" change, and your health will change along with it. The changes you've made in the past four weeks will have major beneficial implications for the rest of your life.

Step back and review all of the changes you've made—and congratulate yourself. Your support team can provide this for you as well (it's okay to tell the members exactly what you'd like them to say—you can even write it down for them).

Take a moment to review your symptom list and see what changes you can note already. Celebrate each improvement, no matter how small. Remember that chronic health problems typically don't improve on their own—they just keep getting a little worse—so each improvement can be looked at as one of your own little miracles.

Congratulations! And remember—what it takes to become clean, green, and lean, it takes to stay clean, green, and lean.

CHAPTER 8

Clean, Green, and Lean Recipes

This chapter contains a selection of delicious and healthy recipes for breakfast, lunch, and dinner from my own kitchen. And as an added bonus, they are *all* gluten free.

For wheat- and gluten-free cooking, you can make the following substitutions for wheat flour. Flour density depends on what the flour is made of, so this list also includes the adjusted amount needed to be equivalent to 1 cup of wheat flour.

1 cup of wheat flour equals:
⅞ cup rice flour
½ cup arrowroot starch
⅝ cup potato starch flour
¾ cup tapioca starch
¾ cup spelt flour (contains gluten)
1 cup corn flour
1 cup teff flour (no gluten)
¾–⅞ cup soy flour

For thickening sauces or gravies: 1 tablespoon flour = ½ tablespoon potato, tapioca, rice, or arrowroot starch.

Look for the gluten-free section in the grocery store, or for gluten-free products mixed in with regular products.

Buckwheat is not wheat. It is not even a grain. You can use buckwheat flour for baking muffins, biscuits, and pancakes. Mixing the gluten- and wheat-free flours when baking is a great idea.

Bon appétit!

Breakfast

Island Smoothie
(Serves 1)

- 1½ cups organic unfiltered apple juice
- 1 ounce Mitogenx Liquid Life (equals 3½ pounds of fruits and vegetables)
- 2 scoops Mitogenx Amino ICG protein powder
- ½ cup frozen pineapple
- ½ cup frozen mango
- 1 banana, sliced
- ice as needed

Mix all of the ingredients together in a blender; add ice for desired consistency.

Apple and Pear Breakfast Smoothie
(Serves 1)

- 1½ cups unfiltered organic apple juice
- 1 ounce Mitogenx Liquid Life (equals 3½ pounds of fruits and vegetables)
- 2 scoops Mitogenx Amino ICG protein powder
- ¾ cup organic apples, diced
- ¾ cup organic pears, diced
- ice as needed

Mix all of the ingredients together in a blender; add ice for desired consistency.

Dr. Crinnion's Berry Wonderful Breakfast
(Serves 1)

> 1½ cups organic unfiltered apple juice
> 1 ounce Mitogenx Liquid Life (equals 3½ pounds of fruits and
>   vegetables)
> 2 scoops Mitogenx Amino ICG protein powder
> ½ cup frozen organic blueberries
> ½ cup frozen organic strawberries
> ice as needed

Mix all of the ingredients together in a blender; add ice for desired consistency.

Fruit and Cottage Cheese
(Serves 1)

> ½ cup organic strawberries (frozen or fresh)
> ½ cup organic blueberries (frozen or fresh)
> ½ cup organic peaches (frozen or fresh)
> ½ cup organic or U.S.-grown grapes
> 1 cup organic low-fat cottage cheese
> roasted macadamia nuts or cashews, whole or halved

Fill a bowl with fruit and top with cottage cheese. Sprinkle the macadamia nuts or cashews on top.

Fruit, Yogurt, and Granola
(Serves 2)

> 1 organic apple, cut into chunks
> 1 banana, cut into slices
> 2 cups watermelon, cut into chunks (can substitute 2 cups organic pear
>   depending on seasonal availability)
> 2 cups organic low-fat plain yogurt
> 1 cup gluten-free granola

Place the fruit in two bowls. Add 1 cup of the yogurt to each bowl and top with granola.

Quinoa, Fruit, and Nut Cereal
(Serves 4)

4 cups water
2 cups gluten-free quinoa
½ cup walnuts, chopped
1 teaspoon cinnamon
¼ teaspoon nutmeg
¼ cup dried cranberries
¼ cup dried blueberries
1 organic pear, diced
rice, almond, or soy milk
honey to taste

In a small saucepan, bring the water to a low boil. Add the quinoa, walnuts, cinnamon, nutmeg, cranberries, blueberries, and pear and simmer until the water has evaporated. Top with the milk of your choice and honey to taste.

Irish Oatmeal with Fruit and Nuts
(Serves 2)

4 cups water
1 cup steel-cut Irish oats
⅛ cup pecans
½ organic apple, diced
⅛ cup dates, raisins, or dried cranberries
1 scoop Mitogenx Amino ICG protein powder
¼ cup rice, almond, or soy milk
1 teaspoon honey or organic brown sugar

Bring the water to a boil in a small saucepan. Add the oats and stir. Reduce the heat to simmer and let cook for 30 minutes. Remove from the heat; add the pecans, diced apple, and your dried fruit of choice. Pour the mixture into a bowl and let cool a few minutes. Add the protein powder and stir. Top with the milk of your choice and add honey or brown sugar to taste.

Scrambled Eggs with Gluten-Free Toast and Fruit
(Serves 2)

> ½ teaspoon organic olive oil
> 4 organic eggs
> organic shredded cheese
> salt and pepper to taste
> 2 slices gluten-free bread
> organic fruit spread
> 2 cups organic strawberries (fresh or frozen)

Grease a small sauté pan with olive oil. Crack the eggs into the pan and scramble over medium heat; sprinkle the cheese over the eggs and melt; add salt and pepper to taste. Toast the bread and top with the fruit spread. Serve strawberries on the side.

Gluten-Free Apple Cinnamon Pancakes with Turkey Bacon
(Serves 2)

> 1 tablespoon organic butter
> ½ cup organic apples, diced
> ½ cup soy flour
> ½ cup brown rice flour
> 1 teaspoon cinnamon
> dash salt
> 1 teaspoon baking powder
> 1 cup rice or soy milk
> 1 organic brown egg
> 1 teaspoon honey
> 2 tablespoons walnut oil
> maple syrup to taste (optional)
> fruit topping (optional)
> 6 slices turkey bacon

In a small sauté pan, melt the butter and stir in the diced apples. Sauté 2 to 3 minutes or until the apples are soft. Set aside. In a medium bowl, add the flour, cinnamon, salt, and baking powder. Mix well and set aside. In another medium bowl, add the rice or soy milk, egg, honey, and 1 tablespoon of the walnut oil. Mix together. Pour the wet mixture into the dry mixture and stir into a moist and lumpy batter. Fold in the sautéed apples. Grease the skillet with 1 tablespoon of the walnut oil and heat. Add the batter to the hot skillet and flip the pancakes only after bubbles appear on the surface. The pancakes should be golden brown. Add maple syrup or a fruit topping of your choice and serve with the turkey bacon after microwaving per the package directions.

Mushroom, Spinach, and Cheese Omelet with Whole-Grain Gluten-Free Toast
(Serves 2)

    1 teaspoon organic olive oil
    ½ cup mushrooms, diced
    ½ cup organic frozen spinach
    4 organic eggs, beaten
    dash salt and pepper
    ¼ cup organic shredded cheese
    2 slices whole-grain gluten-free bread
    2 teaspoons organic fruit preserves

In a small sauté pan, heat the oil and add the mushrooms and spinach, stirring often for 3–4 minutes. Add the beaten eggs and let them set over medium heat. Add a dash of salt and black pepper. When the eggs appear to be mostly cooked, add the shredded cheese and melt. Fold half of the egg preparation over onto itself and cut it in half to serve. Toast the bread and top with the fruit preserves.

Broccoli and Cheese Frittata
(Serves 4)

    2 teaspoons organic olive oil
    2 cups broccoli, chopped
    8 organic eggs
    salt and pepper to taste
    ½ cup organic Monterey Jack cheese
    1 cup organic strawberries

Preheat the oven to broil. In a small sauté pan, add about 1 teaspoon of the olive oil. Stir in 2 cups of the chopped broccoli and cook about 8 minutes over medium heat. Grease an oven-safe skillet with the remaining teaspoon of the organic olive oil. Add the eggs and whisk, cooking over medium heat. Add the cooked broccoli and salt and pepper to taste, continuing to heat until the eggs begin to set. Sprinkle the cheese over the eggs and place the skillet in the oven for about 3–4 minutes or until slightly brown. Let cool, then cut into slices and serve with the strawberries on the side.

Veggie Breakfast Burritos
(Serves 2)

> ½ teaspoon organic olive oil
> 1 organic bell pepper, sliced
> 4 mushrooms, sliced
> 4 organic eggs
> 1 small tomato, diced
> ¼ cup black olives, sliced
> salt and pepper to taste
> 1 jalapeno, sliced, if heat is desired
> 4 corn tortillas
> 4 teaspoons organic Monterey Jack cheese

In a small sauté pan, add the olive oil, bell pepper, and mushrooms. Cook for about 5 minutes. Using a whisk, beat the eggs and add to the sauté pan. Scramble the mixture and add in the tomato, black olives, salt and pepper to taste, and jalapeno, if desired. Heat each corn tortilla for about 15 seconds in the microwave and spoon the egg mixture onto the tortillas. Sprinkle 1 teaspoon of the cheese over the eggs in each tortilla shell and roll them up.

Scrambled Eggs, Tofu, and Broccoli
(Serves 2)

> 1 teaspoon organic olive oil
> 1 cup broccoli, chopped
> 6 ounces firm tofu, diced
> tamari (wheat-free soy sauce)

Spike or other all-purpose seasoning
4 organic eggs
1 cup organic or U.S.-grown grapes

In a sauté pan, add the olive oil and broccoli. Cook over medium heat for about 7 minutes, stirring often. Add the tofu to the pan and drizzle with the tamari and Spike seasoning. In a small bowl, whisk the eggs and then pour them into the sauté pan with the broccoli and tofu. Stir often until the eggs become scrambled. Serve immediately with the grapes on the side.

Veggie Benedict
(Serves 2)

organic olive oil
1 zucchini, diced
1 tomato, diced
1 cup organic frozen spinach, chopped
¼ cup black olives, sliced
Spike or other all-purpose seasoning
½ teaspoon dried rosemary
4 organic eggs
2 gluten-free English muffins, cut in half
¼ cup organic mozzarella cheese

In a small sauté pan, drizzle the olive oil. Add the zucchini, tomato, spinach, and black olives. Sprinkle the Spike seasoning and rosemary over the vegetables and sauté for about 5 minutes over medium heat. Fill a frying pan with water and bring it to a low boil. Poach the eggs in the water for about 4 minutes or to the desired hardness of the yolk. Toast the English muffins. Spoon the vegetable mixture onto the English muffin halves and top with a poached egg. Sprinkle the cheese over the eggs and serve.

Canadian Bacon, Green Pepper, and Onion Quiche
(Serves 4–6)

1 gluten-free pie crust (available at local health food stores)
6 ounces lean Canadian bacon
½ teaspoon organic olive oil

1 organic green pepper, diced

½ yellow onion, diced

1½ cups egg white substitute

½ cup soy or rice milk

1 cup organic low-fat mozzarella cheese, shredded

¼ teaspoon salt

¼ teaspoon black pepper

dash ground nutmeg

Preheat the oven to 450°F. Cover the pie crust with aluminum foil and bake for approximately 10 minutes. Remove the crust from the oven and set aside. Reduce the heat in the oven to 325°F. In a small sauté pan, heat the Canadian bacon over medium heat for about 2 minutes on each side. Remove from the heat and cut into small pieces. Add the olive oil to the sauté pan and throw in the green pepper and onion, stirring constantly. The pepper and onion are done when they appear soft. In a large mixing bowl, add the egg white substitute, milk, cheese, Canadian bacon, green pepper and onion, salt, black pepper, and nutmeg. Mix them together. Pour the mixture into the previously heated pie crust and bake at 325°F for 35–40 minutes or until a knife comes clean after testing the center. Let cool about 15 minutes before serving. This dish can be made the day before and refrigerated.

Egg-White Omelet with Gluten-Free Cinnamon Raisin Toast

(Serves 2)

½ teaspoon organic olive oil

½ organic red bell pepper, diced

½ cup mushrooms, sliced

¼ yellow onion, diced

½ cup frozen organic spinach

1½ cups egg white substitute

dash garlic salt

dash pepper

dash dried dill weed

2 ounces organic low-fat mozzarella cheese, shredded

2 pieces gluten-free cinnamon raisin bread (available at local health food stores)

In a sauté pan, add the olive oil, red bell pepper, mushrooms, onion, and frozen spinach. Cook over medium heat for about 5–7 minutes or until the vegetables soften. Pour the egg white substitute over the vegetables in the sauté pan. Add a dash of garlic salt, pepper, and dill weed. Let the egg mixture begin to solidify as it cooks, then sprinkle the cheese into the pan. Flip one side of the eggs onto itself and continue cooking for another 2 minutes. Cut the omelet in half and serve on two plates. Toast the cinnamon raisin bread and serve one piece per plate.

Gluten-Free Pecan Pancakes, Protein-Style
(Serves 2)

> 2 cups organic gluten-free pancake and baking mix (available at many grocery stores and local health food stores)
> ⅔ cup soy or rice milk
> ¼ cup egg white substitute
> 2 teaspoons walnut oil
> 2 scoops Amino ICG protein powder
> ½ teaspoon ground cinnamon
> 1 teaspoon vanilla extract
> ½ cup pecans (raw or roasted), chopped
> 1 cup organic apple or other fruit sauce

In a large mixing bowl, add the pancake mix, milk, egg white substitute, 1 teaspoon of the walnut oil, protein powder, cinnamon, vanilla, and pecans. Stir the ingredients together well. More or less milk can be added depending on the preferred thickness of the pancakes. Using a griddle or flat pan, grease with the remaining teaspoon of the walnut oil and let the pan get very hot before adding the batter. Flip the pancakes when bubbles appear while cooking. Top with the fruit sauce and serve.

Hard-Boiled Eggs, Fruit Salad, and Toast
(Serves 1)

> water
> 2 organic eggs
> salt and pepper to taste
> 1 cup blueberries
> 1 cup organic strawberries

1 cup organic grapes

1 5-ounce can light Bartlett pear halves in pear juice concentrate and
    water

1 piece gluten-free cinnamon raisin bread

In a small saucepan, bring the water to a boil and cook the eggs for
about 15 minutes. Rinse the eggs with cold water and peel off the
eggshells. Season with salt and pepper to taste. In a medium mixing
bowl, add the blueberries, strawberries, grapes, and pears with juice.
Mix them together. (There will be enough fruit salad left over to
refrigerate for later.) Toast the cinnamon raisin bread and serve with
egg and fruit salad.

Fresh Pineapple, Cottage Cheese, and Almonds
(Serves 2)

4 cups fresh pineapple, cubed

2 cups organic low-fat cottage cheese

4 tablespoons slivered almonds

Divide the pineapple and cottage cheese into two bowls. Top with the
slivered almonds and serve.

Protein Mango Smoothie with Yogurt
(Serves 1)

1 cup organic low-fat plain yogurt

1 cup frozen organic mango

1 cup organic apple juice

2 scoops Amino ICG protein powder

ice

In a blender, add the yogurt, mango, apple juice, and protein powder.
Blend and add ice to the desired consistency.

Sunrise Apple Salad and Turkey Bacon
(Serves 1)

3 slices turkey bacon

1 cup organic low-fat plain yogurt

1 organic apple, diced

¼ cup dried cranberries and blueberries

2 teaspoons raw slivered almonds

2 teaspoons macadamia nuts

Cook the turkey bacon per package directions. In a bowl, combine the yogurt, apple, and dried berries. Top with the nuts and serve with the turkey bacon on the side.

Protein-Style Oatmeal with Nuts and Fruit
(Serves 2)

1 cup organic oatmeal

½ cup dried cranberries, blueberries, apricots, raisins, or prunes

½ cup raw or roasted pecans and walnuts, chopped

2 scoops Amino ICG protein powder

½ cup soy or rice milk

2 teaspoons honey

Prepare the oatmeal according to the package directions. While the oats are cooking, stir in the dried fruit and nuts. Place the oatmeal in two bowls. Let cool before adding the protein powder and milk. Sweeten with honey as desired.

Breakfast Sandwich to Go
(Serves 2)

1 gluten-free English muffin cut in half (available at local health food stores)

2 ounces lean Canadian bacon, precooked

½ teaspoon organic olive oil

1 cup egg white substitute

2 ounces low-fat organic cheese of choice

Toast the English muffin halves, place them on two plates, and top them with the Canadian bacon. In a small sauté pan, add the olive oil and scramble the egg white substitute. Sprinkle the cheese on top of the eggs and allow it to melt. Place the eggs and cheese on top of the English muffin halves and enjoy.

Nourishing Granola with Milk and Berries
(Serves 1)

> 1 cup Bakery on Main gluten-free granola, flavor of choice
> 1 cup organic soy, rice, or almond milk
> ½ cup fresh or frozen blueberries
> ½ cup fresh or frozen organic strawberries

Pour the granola in a bowl and add your milk of choice and the berries.

Egg-White Omelet with Mushrooms, Havarti, and Dill
(Serves 2)

> ½ teaspoon organic olive oil
> 1 cup mushrooms, sliced
> 1½ cups egg white substitute
> 2 ounces light havarti cheese, cubed
> ⅛ cup fresh dill, finely chopped
> 2 pieces gluten-free herb bread (available at local health food stores)

In a small sauté pan, add the olive oil and mushrooms. Sauté over medium heat for about 5 minutes or until the mushrooms become soft. Pour in the egg white substitute and allow the eggs to set as they cook. Toss the cheese and dill on top of the eggs. Flip the omelet over on itself when the edges appear cooked. Cut in half. Toast the bread and serve the omelet on two plates along with the toasted herb bread.

Energy-Boosting Smoothie
(Serves 1)

> ½ cup watermelon, cubed
> ½ cup pineapple, fresh or frozen
> ½ cup mango, fresh or frozen
> ½ cup organic strawberries, fresh or frozen
> 1 cup organic apple juice (use 2 cups if it is too thick for you with just 1 cup)
> 2 scoops Amino ICG protein powder
> 2 ounces Liquid Life
> ice

Place the ingredients in a blender and add ice to the desired consistency. Drink and enjoy.

Breakfast Scramble with Sweet Potato Hash Browns
(Serves 2)

2 cups shredded sweet potatoes, peeled
¼ teaspoon cinnamon
¼ teaspoon nutmeg
¼ teaspoon salt
1 tablespoon organic butter, melted
8 ounces lean Canadian bacon, precooked and diced
½ cup organic green bell pepper, diced
¼ cup onion, diced
½ cup mushrooms, sliced
1 teaspoon organic olive oil

In a small bowl, mix the sweet potatoes, cinnamon, nutmeg, salt, and melted butter. Add the mixture to a large heated sauté pan and cook over medium heat for about 10 minutes. Stir in the Canadian bacon, green bell pepper, onion, mushrooms, and olive oil. Sauté the mixture for approximately 10 more minutes or until tender. Serve on two plates.

Scrambled Egg Whites, Grits, and Turkey Bacon
(Serves 2)

½ teaspoon organic olive oil
1½ cups egg white substitute
Spike or other all-purpose seasoning
4 slices turkey bacon
½ cup Quaker Instant Grits
dash salt and pepper
2 1-teaspoon portions organic butter (one for each bowl)

In a small sauté pan, add the olive oil and egg white substitute. Scramble the eggs to desired consistency and season with Spike or other all-purpose seasoning. Microwave the turkey bacon for about 20–30 seconds or until warm. Make the grits according to the package directions, adding the salt, pepper, and butter once the grits are cooked. Serve the eggs, bacon, and grits on two plates and enjoy.

Homemade Gluten-Free Carrot and Nut Muffins with Yogurt and Fruit
(Serves 2)

> 4 cups gluten-free baking mix (available at many grocery and health food stores)
> 2 teaspoons ground cinnamon
> 2 teaspoons baking powder
> 2 teaspoons xanthan gum
> 1 cup shredded carrots
> 1 cup walnuts, chopped
> ½ cup organic raisins
> 2 organic eggs
> ½ cup walnut oil
> ½ cup water
> 2 cups blueberries
> 2 cups organic grapes
> 2 cups organic low-fat plain yogurt

Preheat the oven to 350°F. In a large mixing bowl, add the baking mix, cinnamon, baking powder, and xanthan gum, and mix them together. In another bowl, add the carrots, walnuts, raisins, eggs, walnut oil, and water, and mix them together well. Slowly pour the liquids into the bowl with the dry ingredients and stir. Grease a muffin pan with a small amount of walnut oil. Bake 15–20 minutes or until a toothpick comes clean from the center of the muffins. Makes twelve muffins.

In two bowls, add the blueberries and grapes, and top with the yogurt. Serve with a muffin on the side. Store the remaining muffins in the refrigerator or freeze for later use.

Lunch

Easy Chicken Salad over Greens
(Serves 2)

> 1 10-ounce can white chicken in spring water
> 2 tablespoons organic light mayonnaise

1 organic apple, diced
¼ cup organic or U.S.-grown grapes
small handful chopped walnuts
salt and pepper to taste
2 cups organic greens per person
8 gluten-free crackers (such as rice crackers)
2 tablespoons red raspberry vinaigrette

Drain the canned chicken and place in a bowl. Add the mayonnaise, apple, grapes, and walnuts. Sprinkle with salt and pepper to taste. Place the chicken salad over the greens and pour the raspberry vinaigrette over it to taste. Serve with the gluten-free crackers.

Bunless Turkey Burger and Mashed Sweet Potatoes
(Serves 4)

Sweet Potatoes
3 large sweet potatoes
3 teaspoons organic butter
1 teaspoon cinnamon
dash nutmeg
¼ cup orange juice
dash salt

Burger
1¼ pounds lean ground turkey
¼ cup chopped cilantro
¼ cup chopped organic bell pepper
½ cup chopped organic celery
1 organic brown egg
2 tablespoons fruit preserves, preferably orange, apricot, or raspberry
1 teaspoon spicy brown mustard
salt and pepper to taste
4 cups organic mixed salad greens
4 half-teaspoons olive oil (one for each individual salad)
4 half-teaspoons balsamic vinegar

Preheat the oven to 425°F. Wash the sweet potatoes and pierce with a fork. Wrap each potato in aluminum foil and cook for 65–75 minutes or until the potatoes are soft. Remove the skin of the potatoes with a fork, and place the potatoes, butter, cinnamon, nutmeg, orange juice, and salt in a large bowl. Mash together and set aside.

In another bowl, add the lean ground turkey, cilantro, bell pepper, celery, egg, fruit preserves, mustard, salt, and pepper. Mix well. Form the mixture into four patties. Grill for about 20 minutes. (Note: The patties may look as if they'll fall apart, but after cooking for a few minutes, they'll hold together nicely.) Serve the burgers with the mashed sweet potatoes and a small green salad dressed with olive oil and balsamic vinegar.

Salmon Spread and Mixed Greens
(Serves 2)

> 1 7½-ounce can Vital Choice Wild Red salmon
> 1 tablespoon organic light mayonnaise
> 1 tablespoon sweet pickle relish
> ¼ cup organic celery, chopped
> dash black pepper
> 4 cups organic mixed salad greens
> 2 half-teaspoons olive oil (one for each individual salad)
> 2 half-teaspoons balsamic vinegar
> 8 rice crackers

In a medium bowl, add the salmon after removing the bones. Stir in the mayonnaise, relish, celery, and black pepper. Serve over the mixed greens and add desired salad dressing. Serve with the rice crackers.

Baked Salmon Salad
(Serves 2)

> 2 teaspoons organic olive oil
> pinch dill
> pinch basil
> pinch lemon pepper
> 2 6-ounce portions wild Alaskan salmon
> organic light Italian salad dressing
> organic mixed salad greens
> 1½ cups organic frozen blueberries
> pine nuts

1 yellow squash
organic olive oil
pinch salt and pepper
dash tamari (wheat-free soy sauce)
12 asparagus stalks
water
red raspberry vinaigrette or other salad dressing of choice

Preheat the oven to 325°F. Grease a 9-inch-square baking dish with 1 teaspoon of the olive oil, sprinkle the salmon with the dill, basil, and lemon pepper, and then place the salmon in the dish. Pour the light Italian dressing over the fish and place in the oven for 25–30 minutes or until the salmon flakes easily with a fork. Spread the salad greens over two plates and add the blueberries and pine nuts. Rinse the yellow squash and slice before placing it in a small sauté pan. Add the rest of the olive oil, salt and pepper, and tamari.

The asparagus can be steamed or steeped after rinsing. To steep, place the stalks in a single layer in a frying pan. Sprinkle the asparagus with a pinch of salt and pour very hot water (from a tea kettle) into the pan until the water level reaches no more than halfway up the asparagus. Cover the frying pan with a lid and turn the burner to high to let some water boil off (do not let all of the water boil off).

When the salmon is ready, use a fork and spatula to remove the skin. Place the squash, asparagus, and salmon over the salad greens when ready. Dress with the raspberry vinaigrette or another salad dressing of your choice.

Fruit Salad Topped with Yogurt
(Serves 2)

2 cups organic strawberries (fresh or frozen)
1 cup organic blueberries (fresh or frozen)
1 cup organic or U.S.-grown grapes
1 banana, sliced
½ cup organic apple juice
1 teaspoon lime juice
2 cups organic plain yogurt
2 tablespoons slivered almonds

In a large bowl, mix the strawberries, blueberries, grapes, banana, apple juice, and lime juice. Spoon the fruit mixture into two bowls. Add 1 cup of the yogurt to each bowl and top with the slivered almonds.

Turkey BLT and Fruit
(Serves 2)

> 8 turkey bacon strips
> 4 slices gluten-free whole-grain bread
> organic light mayonnaise
> 1 organic tomato, sliced
> organic lettuce, shredded
> dash salt and pepper
> 1 cup organic strawberries, fresh or frozen, sliced
> 1 cup organic peaches, fresh or frozen
> 1 cup mango slices, fresh or frozen
> 1 tablespoon honey
> 1 teaspoon lime juice

Cook the bacon in a microwave according to the package directions. Toast the bread slices, then spread the mayonnaise on the toast. Add the bacon, tomato, lettuce, salt, and pepper.

In a small bowl, add the strawberries, peaches, and mango. Drizzle the honey and lime juice over the fruit and stir gently. Spoon into two bowls.

Mediterranean Salad with Grilled Chicken
(Serves 2)

> 8 ounces organic chicken breast
> organic light Italian dressing
> 2 tablespoons rosemary, fresh or dried
> 1 large ripe tomato
> 2 2-ounce portions fresh mozzarella cheese
> ½ cup fresh basil leaves
> 4 tablespoons organic olive oil
> 2 tablespoons balsamic vinegar
> salt and pepper to taste

Preheat the oven to 350°F. Marinate the chicken breast with the Italian dressing. Sprinkle the rosemary on the chicken and place in the oven for about 30 minutes. Place the tomato, cheese, and basil on two plates. Drizzle the olive oil and balsamic vinegar over each plate. When the chicken is cooked through, cut it in strips and place on top of the salads. Add the salt and pepper to taste.

Shrimp and Avocado Soup
(Serves 4)

> 2 cups frozen medium shrimp, shelled
> Spike seasoning
> dash cayenne pepper
> 10 stalks asparagus, cut into 2-inch sections
> 4 stalks organic celery, chopped
> 1 red onion, sliced
> 4 sprigs cilantro
> 6 cups organic chicken broth
> salt and pepper to taste
> 4 ripe avocados, peeled and chopped

In a small sauté pan, add the frozen shrimp and cook about 5–7 minutes over medium heat. Sprinkle the shrimp with a generous amount of the Spike seasoning and the cayenne pepper. In a large saucepan, add the asparagus, celery, onion, cilantro, chicken broth, and salt and pepper. Simmer uncovered for about 20 minutes. Place the mixture in a food processor along with the avocado and purée. Return the mixture to the saucepan and reheat while stirring in the shrimp. Serve hot.

Mozzarella, Tomato, and Pesto on a Herb Baguette
(Serves 2)

> 2 gluten-free herb baguettes from local health food store
> organic olive oil
> 8 ounces buffalo mozzarella, sliced
> 2 Roma tomatoes, sliced
> 2 teaspoons pesto
> 2 teaspoons macadamia nuts, crushed

salt and pepper to taste
8 basil leaves
1 cup organic blueberries

Preheat the oven to 275°F. Slice both baguettes in half and lay them out on aluminum foil. Drizzle all four pieces of the bread with the olive oil. Let the bread warm for about 15 minutes in the oven. Meanwhile, slice the cheese into about eight large pieces. Also, slice the Roma tomatoes and set aside. Remove the bread from the oven and spread about 1 teaspoon of the pesto and 1 teaspoon of the macadamia nuts on both bottom portions of the baguettes. Top with the cheese and sliced tomatoes. Sprinkle salt and pepper to taste, then add four fresh basil leaves per sandwich. Top with the remaining bread. Cut each sandwich in half and serve with the fresh blueberries on the side.

Healthy Italian Wedding Soup
(Serves 4)

½ package lean ground turkey
4 Jennie-O Italian Turkey Sausage links, sliced
Spike seasoning to taste
1 teaspoon sea salt
1 package gluten-free pasta spirals
8 cups water
32 ounces organic vegetable broth
1 14½-ounce can organic tomatoes
3 cups organic frozen spinach
1 teaspoon onion powder

In a large sauté pan, brown the turkey. Season with the Spike, drain, and set aside. Place the sausage in a sauté pan, season with the Spike, and brown. Add the sea salt to a large pot of water and bring to a boil. Stir in the pasta and cook according to the package directions. Drain the pasta and set aside. In a large soup pot, heat the water and the broth, tomatoes, and spinach. Add the turkey, sausage, and onion powder, and stir until a low boil is attained. Reduce the heat to simmer and stir in the pasta. Cover, simmer for about 30 minutes, and serve.

Easy Turkey Chili
(Serves 2)

  organic olive oil
  8 ounces lean ground turkey
  Spike or other all-purpose seasoning
  1 sweet onion, diced
  1 organic bell pepper, diced
  2 cups water
  1 15-ounce can organic kidney beans
  1 15-ounce can organic black beans
  1 15-ounce can diced tomatoes
  1 teaspoon chili powder
  2 tablespoons Vital Choice Organic Salmon Marinade
  ¼ cup organic shredded cheese
  8 rice crackers or 2 pieces gluten-free French bread

In a large skillet, add the olive oil and brown the turkey over medium heat, seasoning generously with the Spike. Add the onion and bell pepper and cook until tender. In a large pot, add the water, kidney beans, black beans, tomatoes, onion, bell pepper, browned turkey, chili powder, and salmon marinade. Bring the mixture to a boil. Reduce the heat, cover, and simmer for 30 minutes. Top with the cheese and serve with the rice crackers or gluten-free French bread.

Turkey Avocado Wrap
(Serves 2)

  4 corn tortillas
  organic ranch salad dressing
  8 ounces sliced turkey
  1 avocado, peeled and diced
  ¼ cup tomatoes, diced
  4 large basil leaves
  1 cup frozen mango

Layer two corn tortillas on each plate. Spread the ranch dressing on the tortillas. Add the turkey, avocado, tomatoes, and basil leaves. Roll into a wrap and serve with the mango on the side.

Tofu Veggie Wrap
(Serves 2)

> 6 ounces firm tofu, divided into 3-ounce portions
> tamari (wheat-free soy sauce) to taste
> 4 corn tortillas
> 4 tablespoons gluten-free hummus
> ¼ cup organic bell pepper, sliced
> ¼ cup organic mixed greens
> ¼ cup tomatoes, diced
> ¼ cup parsley, chopped fine
> ¼ cup organic plain yogurt

Preheat the oven to 325°F. Place the tofu in a small baking dish and drizzle with the tamari, saturating the tofu. Cook for about 15 minutes. Place two corn tortillas overlapping on each of two plates. Spread the hummus over the tortillas and add the cooked tofu on top. Top the tortillas with the bell pepper, mixed greens, tomatoes, and parsley. Drizzle the yogurt over the vegetables and roll into wraps.

Scrumptious Egg Salad Sandwich with Fruit
(Serves 2)

> 4 organic eggs
> water
> ¼ cup organic celery, diced
> ¼ cup sweet pickle relish
> 1 tablespoon organic low-fat mayonnaise
> 1 teaspoon spicy mustard
> salt and pepper to taste
> 4 pieces gluten-free bread of choice
> organic mixed salad greens
> 1 tomato, sliced
> 1 cup organic grapes
> 1 cup organic strawberries, fresh or frozen (thawed)

Place the eggs in a small saucepan and cover with water. Bring the water to a boil and cook for 4 minutes. Reduce heat to a simmer, cover, and continue cooking for 10 minutes more. Place the eggs under cold water and peel.

In a medium bowl, mash the eggs and add the celery, relish, mayonnaise, mustard, and salt and pepper. Mix together well. Toast the bread before topping with the egg salad, mixed greens, and tomato slices. Serve the grapes and strawberries on the side.

Healthy Chef Salad
(Serves 2)

Easy Homemade Salsa
1 28-ounce can organic diced tomatoes
1 organic green pepper, diced
½ red onion
1½ cups cilantro, chopped
½ cup parsley, chopped
3 organic green onions, chopped
1 teaspoon Spike seasoning or other all-purpose seasoning
1 tablespoon fresh-squeezed lemon juice
1 tablespoon fresh-squeezed lime juice
2 diced jalapenos, optional

Salad
Handful organic mixed salad greens for each person
8 ounces deli smoked turkey breast, chopped
2 ounces organic low-fat mozzarella string cheese, chopped
¼ organic green pepper, diced
½ cup organic carrots, sliced
1 teaspoon organic olive oil
1 teaspoon balsamic vinegar
dash each salt and pepper

To make the salsa, combine the salsa ingredients in a large bowl. Toss together until mixed well. Set aside.

In two bowls, add a handful of mixed salad greens. Top with the smoked turkey, cheese, green pepper, carrots, and 1/4 cup of the homemade salsa. Drizzle the olive oil and balsamic vinegar over the salad and season with the salt and pepper. Store the remaining salsa in the refrigerator for later use.

Chicken Salad with Rice Crackers

(Serves 2)

>   1 10-ounce can shredded white chicken meat in spring water
>   4 teaspoons reduced-fat mayonnaise
>   1 stalk organic celery, chopped
>   ½ organic apple, diced
>   ¼ cup organic red grapes, sliced
>   dash each salt and pepper
>   4 cups organic mixed salad greens
>   1 teaspoon organic olive oil
>   1 teaspoon balsamic vinegar
>   rice crackers

In a medium bowl, mix together well the chicken, mayonnaise, celery, apple, grapes, and salt and pepper. Divide the chicken salad onto two plates. In two bowls, add the salad greens, oil, vinegar, and salt and pepper. Serve the chicken salad with the rice crackers and enjoy the mixed greens on the side.

Tofu BBQ Sandwiches with Vegetables

(Serves 2)

>   1 package extra-firm tofu
>   ¼ cup Annie's Naturals Organic Original BBQ sauce
>   ¼ teaspoon celery salt
>   ¼ teaspoon onion powder
>   ¼ teaspoon garlic powder
>   water
>   ½ cup cauliflower, chopped
>   ½ cup broccoli, chopped
>   ½ cup yellow squash, chopped
>   2 pieces gluten-free herb bread (available at a local health food store)

Preheat the oven to 325°F. In a baking dish, add the tofu, barbecue sauce, celery salt, onion powder, and garlic powder. Mix them together, mashing the tofu. Cook about 15 minutes. In a steamer pan, add about 1 inch of water. Add the cauliflower, broccoli, and yellow squash, and cover. Bring to a boil and allow the vegetables to steam about 15 minutes. Toast the gluten-free bread and place 1 piece on each plate. Top with the barbecued tofu and enjoy the steamed vegetables on the side.

Salmon Salad
(Serves 3)

2 7½-ounce cans Vital Choice Wild Red salmon
2 tablespoons light mayonnaise
1 stalk organic celery, chopped
dash salt
½ teaspoon black pepper
6 cups organic mixed salad greens
12 green olives, sliced
½ organic green bell pepper
½ cup organic carrots, chopped
1½ teaspoons organic olive oil
1½ teaspoons balsamic vinegar

In a medium mixing bowl, carefully add the salmon, removing any small pieces of bone. Add the mayonnaise, celery, salt, and pepper. Stir together. Divide the mixed salad greens among three bowls. Add the green olives, green bell pepper, and carrots to the salad bowls. Top with about 5 ounces each of the salmon salad. Drizzle ½ teaspoon olive oil and ½ teaspoon balsamic vinegar over each salad. Serve and enjoy.

Tofu and Stir-Fry Vegetable Salad
(Serves 2)

3 tablespoons organic olive oil
1 organic yellow bell pepper, sliced
1 organic red bell pepper, sliced
1 cup broccoli, sliced
1 cup cauliflower, sliced
1 cup snow peas
1 cup mushrooms, sliced
1 package extra-firm tofu, sliced
tamari to taste
4 cups organic mixed salad greens

In a wok or large pot, add 2 tablespoons of the olive oil and heat. Carefully toss in the yellow bell pepper, red bell pepper, broccoli, cauliflower, snow peas, and mushrooms. Stir-fry about 5 minutes or until the vegetables appear soft. Add the tofu to the wok with the vegetables and cover the mixture with a generous amount of the tamari. Cook another 2 minutes before removing from the heat. On each of two plates, add the mixed greens. Top with the stir-fry vegetables and tofu. Drizzle ½ teaspoon of the remaining olive oil over each salad and serve.

Grilled Chicken, Cantaloupe, and Pear Salad
(Serves 2)

> 2 organic chicken breasts
> Newman's Own Light Italian Dressing to taste
> dried basil
> 4 cups organic mixed salad greens
> ½ cantaloupe, cubed
> 1 can light Bartlett pear halves in pear juice and water, drained
> 2 tablespoons pine nuts
> Newman's Own Raspberry and Walnut Vinaigrette

Preheat the oven to 350°F. In a large baking dish, arrange the chicken breasts and cover them with the Italian dressing. Sprinkle the dried basil over the chicken and cook for approximately 35 minutes or until the chicken is cooked through. On two plates, arrange the mixed salad greens and top with the cantaloupe and pear. Sprinkle pine nuts over the salad and add one cooked chicken breast per plate. Drizzle the salad with the vinaigrette.

Turkey and Avocado Sandwich with Grapes
(Serves 1)

> 2 slices gluten-free cheese bread (available at a local health food store)
> 1 teaspoon Dijon mustard
> 4–6 ounces smoked deli turkey
> ½ avocado, sliced
> organic mixed greens
> 2 slices tomato
> 1 cup organic green grapes

Toast the bread and spread the Dijon mustard on the bread. Top with the smoked turkey and avocado, and then add the mixed greens and tomato. Serve the organic grapes on the side.

New Orleans–Style Sausage, Beans, and Rice
(Serves 2)

> 1 cup water
> 1 cup organic chicken broth
> dash salt
> 1 cup brown rice, rinsed
> ½ teaspoon organic olive oil
> 2 cups broccoli
> 1 package (approximately 4 links) organic chicken and apple sausage, precooked
> 1 14½-ounce can organic kidney beans
> dash Cajun seasoning, optional

In a medium pot, bring the water and chicken broth to a boil. Add the dash of salt, if desired. Stir in the brown rice, reduce the heat to a simmer, and cover the pot while the rice cooks, about 35–45 minutes, stirring occasionally until all the liquid has evaporated. Meanwhile, in a small sauté pan, add the olive oil and broccoli and stir-fry about 5–7 minutes or until the broccoli appears tender. Remove the broccoli and set aside. Add the sausage links to the sauté pan and heat about 2 minutes. Remove the sausage and slice into ½-inch pieces. When the rice has finished cooking, toss in the sausage, kidney beans, and broccoli. Mix the ingredients together along with the Cajun seasoning, and heat about 5 minutes. Serve in two bowls.

Cottage Cheese with Peaches and Cantaloupe
(Serves 1)

> 1 cup organic low-fat cottage cheese
> 1 cup organic peaches, sliced
> 1 cup cantaloupe, cubed

Add peaches and cantaloupe to a bowl and top with cottage cheese.

Chicken Salad on Mixed Greens with Berries
(Serves 2)

> 2 small organic chicken breasts (approximately 4 ounces each)
> ½ cup Newman's Own Raspberry and Walnut Vinaigrette

4 cups organic mixed salad greens
2 cups blueberries
2 cups raspberries
2 teaspoons organic olive oil
2 teaspoons balsamic vinegar
dash each salt and pepper

Preheat the oven to 350°F. In a baking dish, place the chicken breasts and top with the salad dressing. Cook for 30–35 minutes or until the chicken is cooked through. On two plates, arrange the mixed salad greens, blueberries, and raspberries. Add one chicken breast to each plate and dress the salad with the olive oil and balsamic vinegar. Sprinkle with the salt and pepper to taste.

Shrimp Salad Ooh La La!
(Serves 2)

4 cups organic romaine lettuce, torn
8 ounces frozen, peeled, and cooked shrimp
¼ cup organic red bell pepper, diced
¼ cup tomatoes, diced
½ cup broccoli, chopped
½ cup carrots, shredded
10 green olives, chopped
2 hard-boiled organic eggs, chopped
dash each salt and pepper
¼ cup Annie's Naturals Organic Thousand Island Dressing

On two plates, place the romaine lettuce, shrimp, red bell pepper, tomatoes, broccoli, carrots, green olives, and hard-boiled eggs. Add a dash each of the salt and pepper. Drizzle the salad dressing on top and enjoy.

Peanut Butter and Jelly with Watermelon and Apricot Salad
(Serves 1)

1 cup watermelon, cubed
½ cup apricots, sliced
1 teaspoon pineapple juice
1 teaspoon lime juice

1 teaspoon organic apple juice
2 slices gluten-free bread, flavor of choice
2 tablespoons organic peanut butter
1 tablespoon organic strawberry preserves

In a small bowl, mix together the watermelon, apricots, pineapple juice, lime juice, and apple juice. Toast the gluten-free bread and spread the peanut butter and strawberry preserves on top. Cut the bread in half and enjoy with the fruit salad on the side.

Salmon Salad with Fresh Fruit Salsa
(Serves 2)

Salmon
2 6-ounce portions wild Alaskan salmon
organic light Italian dressing (such as Newman's Own)
dried basil
Vital Choice Organic Salmon Marinade

Salsa
1 cup pineapple chunks, fresh or frozen
1 cup mango, fresh or frozen
1 organic apple, diced
1 cup organic bell peppers, chopped
½ cup organic celery, chopped
½ cup parsley, chopped fine
4 tablespoons lime juice
2 teaspoons honey
salt and pepper to taste
organic mixed salad greens
pine nuts
balsamic vinegar

Preheat the oven to 325°F. Place the salmon in a baking dish and drizzle the salad dressing over both pieces. Sprinkle the salmon with the dried basil and salmon marinade. Cook about 25–30 minutes or until the salmon flakes easily with a fork.

While the salmon is cooking, add the pineapple, mango, apple, bell peppers, celery, parsley, lime juice, honey, and salt and pepper in a large mixing bowl. Toss them together well.

On two plates, spread the salad greens and sprinkle with the pine nuts. Top with the salmon and salsa. Drizzle the balsamic vinegar over the salads and serve.

Teriyaki Salmon Salad
(Serves 2)

> 2 medium portions wild Alaskan salmon (red or silver) (5–6 ounces each)
> ¼ cup organic teriyaki sauce of choice
> dash Vital Choice Organic Salmon Marinade
> 4 cups organic mixed salad greens
> 1 cup fresh pineapple, cubed
> 1 cup frozen organic mango
> 2 tablespoons pine nuts
> 1 teaspoon organic olive oil
> 1 teaspoon balsamic vinegar

Preheat the oven to 325°F. In a baking dish, place the salmon and spoon the teriyaki sauce on top. Sprinkle the salmon marinade on top of the fish. Bake for about 30–35 minutes or until the salmon flakes easily with a fork. On two plates, spread the mixed greens and top with the salmon. Add the pineapple and mango, and sprinkle with the pine nuts. Drizzle the olive oil and balsamic vinegar over the salads and serve.

Dinner

Baked Salmon over Pesto Pasta
(Serves 2)

> 2 6-ounce wild Alaskan salmon fillets
> organic light Italian salad dressing
> 2 teaspoons dried basil
> 1 package rice pasta
> 2 tablespoons pesto
> 2 tablespoons organic olive oil
> 4 cups organic mixed salad greens

2 half-teaspoon portions of olive oil (one for each individual salad)
2 half-teaspoon portions balsamic vinegar

Preheat the oven to 350°F. Place the salmon fillets in a baking dish and generously pour the salad dressing over the salmon. Sprinkle the salmon with the dried basil and cook for 30–35 minutes. Cook the pasta according to the package directions. Drain the pasta, rinse, and place it in a medium mixing bowl. Add the pesto and olive oil to the pasta and mix well. Put the pasta on two plates. Remove the skin from the salmon and place the salmon on top of the pasta. Serve with a small green salad dressed with olive oil and vinegar.

Baked Scallops with Risotto and Artichokes
(Serves 4)

Scallops
1¼ pounds jumbo sea scallops
organic light Italian salad dressing
Vital Choice Organic Salmon Marinade
dried basil
lemon pepper

Risotto
1½ cups arborio rice
½ cup green onion, chopped
1 tablespoon organic olive oil
2 cups water
1 cup organic vegetable broth
½ teaspoon sea salt
dash black pepper
dash garlic powder
half a 14-ounce can artichoke quarters

Preheat the oven to 325°F. Place the sea scallops (thawed, if frozen) in a single layer in a baking dish. Pour a generous amount of the salad dressing over the scallops, ensuring complete coverage. Sprinkle the marinade, dried basil, and lemon pepper over the scallops. Bake for 20–25 minutes.

In a small saucepan, sauté the rice and green onion in the olive oil over medium heat. When the rice begins to brown, add the water and vegetable broth, and bring to a boil. Reduce the heat to a simmer and stir in the sea salt, black pepper, garlic powder, and artichokes. Stir frequently for about 20 minutes, leaving the saucepan uncovered. Spoon the risotto onto plates and top with the scallops.

Turkey Sausage and Peppers over Brown Rice

(Serves 2)

Rice

2 cups water
1 cup organic vegetable broth
dash salt
1½ cups long-grain brown rice

Sausage and Peppers

¾ cup organic sweet orange and red bell peppers, sliced
¼ cup green onions, chopped
2 tablespoons organic olive oil
half a 14-ounce can diced tomatoes
1 teaspoon dried basil
1 teaspoon garlic powder
2 teaspoons dried oregano
2 teaspoons Vital Choice Organic Salmon Marinade
1 pound (about 3–4 links) lean turkey sausage links, diced
¼ cup red wine

In a saucepan, bring the water, vegetable broth, and salt to a boil. Stir in the rice and reduce heat to a simmer. Cover and cook for about 45 minutes or until the water has evaporated.

With 15 minutes remaining in the cooking time for the rice, in a separate pan, sauté the peppers and green onions in 1 tablespoon of the olive oil. Add the tomatoes, basil, garlic powder, oregano, and salmon marinade. Cook, stirring often, for about 10 minutes. In another skillet, sauté the turkey sausage in the remaining 1 tablespoon of the olive oil. As the sausage browns, stir in the red wine and simmer about 5 minutes. Mix the peppers, onions, and tomatoes in with the rice. Serve the rice on plates and top with the turkey sausage.

Rosemary Baked Chicken with Orange Rice and Broccoli

(Serves 2)

> 1 cup water
> 1 cup orange juice
> dash salt
> 1 cup whole-grain brown rice (short or long grain)
> organic olive oil
> 2 8-ounce organic chicken breasts
> ½ cup champagne vinaigrette dressing (available at most grocery stores)
> dried rosemary
> 3–4 cups broccoli
> Spike or other all-purpose seasoning

Preheat the oven to 350°F. In a saucepan, bring the water, orange juice, and salt to a boil. Rinse the rice, then add it to the boiling water and orange juice mixture. Once the liquid resumes boiling, reduce to a simmer. Place the lid on the saucepan and cook, allowing all of the water to boil off (about 40–45 minutes).

Cover the bottom of a 9-inch-square baking dish with the olive oil. Place the chicken breasts in the dish and pour the champagne vinaigrette dressing over the chicken. Sprinkle a generous amount of the rosemary on the chicken. Bake 35 minutes or until the chicken is tender. Wash the broccoli and cut the heads off of the stalks, slicing into quarters. Sprinkle the broccoli with the Spike or other all-purpose seasoning and steam for about 8–10 minutes or until the broccoli is a vibrant green. Serve the chicken over the rice, with the broccoli on the side.

Dr. Crinnion's Excellent Chicken and Vegetable Enchiladas

(Serves 6)

> 5 large mushrooms, sliced
> ½ large sweet onion, diced
> 1 organic bell pepper, diced
> ⅔ cup frozen chopped organic spinach, thawed

1 stalk organic celery, diced

2 tablespoons organic olive oil

1 15-ounce can organic pinto beans

1 14½-ounce can organic diced tomatoes

salt to taste

8 ounces cooked chicken breast, diced

1 sweet potato, cooked and mashed

1 tablespoon tarragon

1 tablespoon marjoram

15 small corn tortillas

1 jar enchilada sauce, mild, medium, or hot

1 cup organic shredded cheese

Preheat the oven to 325°F. In a large frying pan, sauté the mushrooms, onion, bell pepper, spinach, and celery in the olive oil. Turn down the heat on the frying pan. Drain the beans and tomatoes, and add them to the frying pan with the salt. Stir in the chicken, sweet potato, tarragon, and marjoram, and simmer about 10 minutes to combine the flavors, stirring occasionally. Line the bottom of a 3-quart, 13 × 9 × 2–inch baking dish with the corn tortillas. Spoon about half of the cooked mixture on top of the tortillas. Add more tortillas in a second layer and spoon the rest of the mixture on top. Layer the remaining tortillas on top and cover with the enchilada sauce. Sprinkle the cheese over the enchilada sauce. Cover the dish with aluminum foil and bake in the oven for 20 minutes. Use a spatula to serve.

Baked Tofu with Stir-Fried Vegetables over Brown Rice
(Serves 2)

1 cup water

1 cup chicken or vegetable broth

dash salt

1 cup whole-grain brown rice (long or short grain)

1 package tofu (medium to extra firm), cubed

tamari (wheat-free soy sauce)

2 tablespoons organic olive oil

½ organic red bell pepper, chopped

½ organic green bell pepper, chopped

1 cup broccoli, chopped
½ medium sweet onion, diced
1 yellow squash, chopped
5 small mushrooms, chopped
¼ cup cashews
1 teaspoon tarragon
1 teaspoon marjoram

In a saucepan, add the the water, broth, and salt, and bring to a boil. After washing the rice, add it to the boiling liquid. Once the liquid resumes boiling, reduce the heat to a simmer and cover, allowing the liquid to cook off (about 40–45 minutes).

Preheat the oven to 350°F. In a baking dish, add the tofu. Cover the tofu with tamari and bake for about 15 minutes. Add the olive oil to a hot wok or large frying pan. Add the red and green bell pepper, broccoli, onion, squash, and mushrooms, one at a time, coating each new vegetable with a little extra olive oil after adding it to the wok. Throw in the cashews, tamari, a bit more salt, tarragon, and marjoram to the vegetable mixture, and cook about 10 minutes, stirring constantly. Turn the heat down to a simmer and cover, allowing the mixture to cook 5 minutes more. Place the rice on plates and top with the vegetables and tofu.

Gluten-Free Pizza with Turkey Sausage, Peppers, and Mushrooms
(Serves 2)

organic olive oil
2 small gluten-free pizza crusts
dried basil
dried oregano
7 links turkey sausage, diced
1 cup organic red, yellow, and orange peppers, sliced
1 cup mushrooms, sliced
organic shredded mozzarella cheese
4 cups organic mixed salad greens
1 teaspoon olive oil (one for each individual salad)
1 teaspoon balsamic vinegar

Preheat the oven to 325°F. Spread a generous amount of olive oil on the gluten-free pizza crusts. Sprinkle the basil and oregano on both crusts and set aside. In a small sauté pan coated with olive oil, add the sausage links and cook until brown. Drain the sausage and place on a paper towel. Add more olive oil to the pan and stir in the peppers and mushrooms, and sauté about 3–4 minutes. Add the sausage, peppers, and mushrooms to the pizza crusts. Sprinkle a generous amount of the cheese over the other ingredients. Place the pizzas in the oven for about 20 minutes or until the cheese begins to brown slightly. Cool and serve with a small green salad dressed with organic olive oil and balsamic vinegar.

BBQ Chicken with Mashed Butternut Squash and Broccoli Salad
(Serves 2)

BBQ Chicken
2 organic chicken breasts
2 teaspoons organic olive oil
Spike or other all-purpose seasoning
organic barbecue sauce (such as Annie's Naturals)
1 tablespoon dried rosemary

Butternut Squash
1 large butternut squash, halved
organic olive oil
¼ sweet onion, diced
1 tablespoon organic butter
1 teaspoon organic brown sugar
½ cup pecans, roasted and chopped
2 tablespoons parsley, chopped

Broccoli Salad
3 tablespoons organic olive oil
½ teaspoon lime juice
2 tablespoons honey
10 ounces organic broccoli slaw
¼ cup dried cranberries, chopped fine
2 tablespoons slivered almonds

¼ teaspoon sea salt
¼ teaspoon black pepper

Preheat the oven to 350°F. In a small baking dish, place the chicken breasts and rub with 2 teaspoons of the olive oil. Sprinkle the Spike or other all-purpose seasoning over each chicken breast. Cover the chicken with the barbecue sauce and top with the dried rosemary. Bake 30–35 minutes or until the chicken is cooked through.

In another baking dish, place the butternut squash halves and cover with a paper towel. Microwave on high 6 minutes. Let the squash sit a couple of minutes before microwaving on high another 6 minutes. In a large sauté pan, add the olive oil and diced onion. Sauté over medium heat 7–8 minutes or until the onion is golden brown. When the squash has finished microwaving, spoon out the seeds and discard. Using a fork, add the squash to the sauté pan with the onions and add in the butter, brown sugar, and pecans. Stir everything together and serve with the chopped parsley on top.

In a mixing bowl, add 3 teaspoons of the olive oil, lime juice, and honey. Mix them together and add the broccoli slaw, cranberries, and slivered almonds. Stir everything together, add salt and pepper, and serve chilled. This salad can be made the day before.

Salmon and Spinach over Pasta
(Serves 2)

4 cups water
dash salt
1 package gluten-free pasta spirals
1 7½-ounce can Vital Choice Wild Red salmon, bones removed
1 cup frozen organic chopped spinach
1 cup organic plain yogurt
1 tablespoon Vital Choice Organic Salmon Marinade
parmesan cheese, grated

In a large pot, boil the water with the salt. Cook the pasta according to the package directions. Drain the pasta and return it to the pot, stirring in the salmon and spinach. Cook the mixture about 2 minutes. In a medium mixing bowl, add the yogurt and salmon marinade, and mix them together. Add the pasta, salmon, and spinach to the yogurt mixture, stirring well. Top with the cheese and serve warm.

Salmon and Vegetable Tacos
(Serves 2)

   1 organic bell pepper, sliced
   1 sweet onion, sliced
   organic olive oil
   2 7½-ounce cans Vital Choice Wild Red salmon, bones removed
   1 tablespoon Vital Choice Organic Salmon Marinade
   1 can organic pinto beans
   4 corn tortillas
   1 avocado, diced
   1 tomato, diced
   organic shredded cheese
   organic salsa (mild, medium, or hot)
   organic mixed salad greens

In a small sauté pan, sauté the bell pepper and onion in the olive oil about 5 minutes. Add the salmon, then blend in the salmon marinade. Continue to heat the mixture a few minutes, stirring thoroughly. In a small saucepan, heat the pinto beans over medium heat. Microwave the corn tortillas about 15 seconds each to warm. On top of the tortillas, add the salmon, bell pepper, onion, and beans. Top with the avocado, tomato, cheese, and salsa, and serve with the mixed salad greens.

Mushroom, Eggplant, and Swiss Chard Lasagna
(Serves 6–8)

   organic olive oil
   1 eggplant, sliced lengthwise and cut into 1-inch pieces
   4 cups Swiss chard, chopped
   1 package organic brown rice lasagna noodles
   2 cups mushrooms, sliced
   16 ounces organic low-fat cottage cheese
   1 teaspoon organic dried oregano
   1 teaspoon garlic powder

1 tablespoon organic dried basil
2 14½-ounce cans tomato sauce
1 cup organic shredded mozzarella cheese

In a sauté pan, add the olive oil and eggplant, and sauté over medium heat about 5 minutes. Fill a large pot about one-third with water and bring to a boil. Add the Swiss chard to the boiling water, cover, and cook about 10–15 minutes. Drain the chard and set aside. Cook the rice noodles in a large pot according to the package directions, and drain. Preheat the oven to 350°F. In a mixing bowl, add the mushrooms, cottage cheese, oregano, garlic powder, and basil, and stir together. Spread about 1 cup of the tomato sauce on the bottom of a 13 × 9 × 2–inch baking dish. Top the sauce with the rice noodles. Spoon the eggplant and Swiss chard over the noodles, then top with the mixture of cottage cheese, mushrooms, and spices. Repeat this layering process again, and finish with the remaining tomato sauce and a layer of noodles and cheese. Cover the baking dish with aluminum foil and bake 30–35 minutes. Remove the foil and continue to cook 15–20 minutes more or until the top has browned nicely. Cut into portions and serve.

Jammin' Jambalaya
(Serves 4)

2 tablespoons organic olive oil
4 Jennie-O lean Italian sausage links, sliced in ½-inch pieces
1 cup organic sweet bell peppers, sliced
½ cup green onion, diced
½ cup organic celery, diced
2 cups brown rice
4 cups organic chicken broth
¼ teaspoon black pepper
¼ teaspoon cayenne pepper
1 teaspoon thyme
3 bay leaves
4 cups organic mixed salad greens
2 half-teaspoon portions of olive oil (one for each individual salad)
2 half-teaspoon portions balsamic vinegar

In a large pot, drizzle the olive oil, then add the turkey sausage. Cook the sausage until browned over medium heat. Add the bell peppers, green onion, and celery, and sauté about 5 minutes. Stir in the uncooked brown rice, chicken broth, black pepper, cayenne pepper, thyme, and bay leaves. Bring to a boil, then reduce the heat and cover. Cook about 40 minutes, stirring occasionally. Remove the bay leaves and serve with a small green salad dressed with organic olive oil and balsamic vinegar.

Turkey and Artichoke Casserole
(Serves 4)

1 cup water
1 cup organic vegetable broth
dash salt
1 cup brown rice
1 teaspoon organic olive oil
1 cup broccoli, chopped
½ cup organic bell peppers, sliced
½ cup organic carrots, chopped
1 12½-ounce can white chunk turkey
1 14-ounce can quartered artichoke hearts
¾ cup organic rice milk
¾ cup dried cranberries
1 14½-ounce can organic cream of chicken soup

In a small saucepan, bring the water, vegetable broth, and salt to a boil. Add the rice to the boiling water, reduce to a simmer, and cover. Cook about 45 minutes. Preheat the oven to 350°F. In a large skillet, add the olive oil, broccoli, bell peppers, and carrots. Cook over medium heat about 10 minutes. Remove from the heat and stir in the turkey, artichoke hearts, rice milk, cranberries, cream of chicken soup, and cooked rice. Place the mixture in a 13 × 9 × 2–inch baking dish and cover with aluminum foil. Bake 25 minutes, then remove the foil and bake 15–20 minutes more. Remove from the oven and serve.

Bean and Cheese Soft Tacos with Homemade Salsa
(Serves 2)

4 corn tortillas
1 15-ounce can organic pinto beans

1 cup organic low-fat shredded cheese of choice
dash Spike seasoning or taco seasoning
2 cups organic mixed salad greens
Homemade Salsa (see recipe on page 221)

Preheat the oven to 300°F. Place the corn tortillas on individual sheets of aluminum foil. Top with the pinto beans, cheese, and seasoning. Wrap each taco in foil and place them in the oven for approximately 8–10 minutes. Remove the tacos and place them on plates, adding the mixed greens and salsa to each taco. Serve and enjoy.

Salmon with Lemon Butter Sauce and Sautéed Zucchini and Yellow Squash

(Serves 2)

2 tablespoons organic butter
juice of 1 lemon
2 tablespoons organic chives, chopped
⅛ cup organic soy or rice milk
1 teaspoon gluten-free all-purpose flour
dash each salt and pepper
2 wild Alaskan salmon fillets, approximately 4–6 ounces each
½ teaspoon organic olive oil
1 zucchini, sliced
1 yellow squash, sliced
½ teaspoon Spike or other all-purpose seasoning
fresh organic chives

In a small saucepan over medium heat, melt the butter. Stir in the lemon juice, chives, milk, flour, and salt and pepper. Cook until the sauce begins to thicken.

Preheat the oven to 325°F. Place the salmon on aluminum foil and coat with the lemon butter sauce. Cook 30–35 minutes or until the fish flakes easily with a fork. Meanwhile, add the olive oil to a small sauté pan. Throw in the zucchini and squash, and sprinkle with the Spike seasoning. Sauté about 10–15 minutes or until the desired consistency is reached. Remove the fish from the oven and sprinkle the chives on top. Serve with the vegetables.

Spaghetti Squash with Ground Turkey Tomato Sauce
(Serves 3–4)

> 1 spaghetti squash, halved lengthwise
> 1 package lean ground turkey
> Spike seasoning to taste
> 1 jar Newman's Own Sockarooni Sauce
> 2 cups organic mixed salad greens
> 1 teaspoon organic olive oil
> 1 teaspoon balsamic vinegar
> dash each salt and pepper

Preheat the oven to 350°F. Fill a shallow baking dish with about 2 inches of water. Place the squash halves face down in the dish and bake about 25 minutes. After cooling, use a fork to discard the seeds and loosen the spaghetti strands. Place the squash in a large bowl and set aside. Brown the ground turkey in a small pan while adding the Spike seasoning to taste. Heat the Sockarooni Sauce in a large pot and add the turkey. Spoon the meat sauce over the spaghetti squash and serve with salad greens topped with olive oil, balsamic vinegar, and salt and pepper.

Vinaigrette Chicken with Broccoli
(Serves 2)

> 2 medium organic chicken breasts
> ¼ cup Newman's Own Light Italian Dressing
> 1 teaspoon Vital Choice Organic Salmon Marinade
> 3 cups broccoli
> 1 tablespoon tamari
> dash black pepper

Preheat the oven to 350°F. In a baking dish, place the chicken breasts and cover with the salad dressing. Sprinkle the chicken with the salmon marinade. Cook about 35 minutes or until the chicken is cooked through. Fill a steamer pot with a couple of inches of water. Add the broccoli, drizzle with the tamari, and add a dash of black pepper. Cover and steam about 15–20 minutes or to desired consistency. Serve the broccoli alongside the chicken and enjoy. This dish may be served with mixed greens and olive oil and balsamic vinegar, if desired.

Turkey Burgers BBQ-Style with Sweet Potato Baked Fries

(Serves 3–4)

1 pound lean ground turkey
¼ cup Annie's Naturals Organic Original BBQ Sauce
6 green onions, diced
1 cup mushrooms, sliced
Spike seasoning
2 medium sweet potatoes, sliced into ½-inch pieces
organic olive oil
sea salt to taste
organic mixed salad greens
1 large tomato, sliced

In a large bowl, add the ground turkey, barbecue sauce, green onions, mushrooms, and Spike seasoning. Stir the mixture together, then form three to four burger patties. Set aside on a plate.

Preheat the oven to 350°F. Wash the sweet potatoes. Place a layer of aluminum foil on a baking sheet. Arrange the sweet potato slices in a single layer on the sheet and drizzle with the olive oil. Sprinkle with the sea salt and cook about 30–35 minutes.

Meanwhile, add the burger patties to a cool skillet. Pan broil the burgers over medium heat for 5–6 minutes per side, depending on the desired degree of doneness. Serve the burgers on plates and top with the greens and sliced tomato. Enjoy the sweet potato slices on the side.

Seared Ham, Steamed Carrots, and Broccoli Slaw

(Serves 2)

6 ounces rice noodles, cooked
1 package organic broccoli slaw
4 ounces slivered almonds
6 green onions, diced
⅓ cup organic olive oil
3 packets Splenda
¼ cup brown rice vinegar
½ teaspoon salt

½ teaspoon black pepper

½ teaspoon Spike or other all-purpose seasoning

1½ cups organic carrots

2 ¼-inch premium ham steaks from the deli (deli section at most grocery stores can cut this for you)

1 teaspoon brown sugar

dash ground cinnamon

2 teaspoons organic butter

Cook the rice noodles according to package directions. Drain and rinse the noodles and add to a large mixing bowl. Add the broccoli slaw, slivered almonds, green onions, olive oil, Splenda, brown rice vinegar, salt, pepper, and Spike seasoning. Mix them together and refrigerate. For the best flavor, prepare the day before.

In steamer pot, add the carrots, cover, and cook over medium heat about 30 minutes or until the desired consistency is reached. In a small sauté pan, sear the ham about 2 minutes on each side. Serve the ham on two plates and add a sprinkling of brown sugar, cinnamon, and butter to the carrots. The broccoli slaw can be served warm or cold.

Teriyaki Noodles, Scallops, and Vegetable Stir-Fry
(Serves 3–4)

dash salt

1 package rice spaghetti noodles

3 tablespoons organic olive oil

2 cups broccoli

½ cup water chestnuts

1 cup carrots, diced

1 yellow squash, sliced

12–16 large fresh or frozen sea scallops

1 jar teriyaki sauce of choice

1 cup fresh cilantro, chopped

Fill a large pot halfway with water, add the salt, and bring to a boil. Add the rice noodles and cook according to the package directions. Drain and rinse the noodles and set them aside. In a wok, add the olive oil. When the oil is hot, add the broccoli, water chestnuts, carrots, and yellow squash. Cook the vegetables about 3–4 minutes, then toss in the scallops. Add the teriyaki sauce and mix the ingredients together well. Cook about 5 more minutes. Serve the rice noodles on plates and top with the vegetables and scallops. Sprinkle with the fresh cilantro and enjoy.

Wild Alaskan Salmon in Fruit Sauce with Brown Rice and Broccoli
(Serves 2)

½ cup organic apple juice
1½ cups water
dash salt
1 cup brown rice, rinsed
2 tablespoons pine nuts
2 medium portions wild red or silver Alaskan salmon
1 jar organic apple/apricot sauce or other fruit sauce of choice
dash Vital Choice Organic Salmon Marinade
2 cups broccoli, chopped

Preheat the oven to 325°F. In a small saucepan, bring the apple juice, water, and salt to a boil. Pour in the brown rice, cover, and reduce the heat to a simmer. Cook about 35–45 minutes or until all of the liquid has been absorbed. Add the pine nuts to the rice when the cooking time is nearly complete.

In a baking dish, place the salmon fillets and spread the fruit sauce on top. Sprinkle the fish with the salmon marinade and bake in the oven about 30–35 minutes or until the fish flakes easily with a fork.

Fill a steamer pot with a couple of inches of water. Add the broccoli, cover and steam about 15–20 minutes or to desired consistency. Serve the salmon over the rice.

Scallops with Asparagus and Brown Rice
(Serves 3–4)

12–16 large fresh or frozen sea scallops
champagne vinaigrette dressing (available at most grocery stores)
dash dried basil

2 cups water
2 cups organic chicken broth
dash salt
2 cups brown rice
20 stalks asparagus, rinsed
4 half-teaspoons parmesan cheese

Preheat the oven to 325°F. In a baking dish, arrange the scallops in a single layer. Drizzle the vinaigrette on top of the scallops before sprinkling with the dried basil. Set aside and allow the scallops to marinate. In a medium saucepan, bring the water and chicken broth with the salt to a boil. Pour in the brown rice and reduce the heat to a simmer, stirring occasionally. Cook the rice covered 35–45 minutes or until all of the liquid has been absorbed. Allow about 15 minutes before the rice is finished to bake the scallops in the oven. Meanwhile, place the asparagus in a steamer pot and steam for 15–20 minutes on high heat. Serve the rice with the scallops on top and the asparagus on the side. Sprinkle the cheese over the asparagus.

Turkey, Spinach, and Mushroom Lasagna
(Serves 6–8)

1 package brown rice lasagna noodles
1 package lean ground turkey
Spike or other all-purpose seasoning
1 teaspoon organic olive oil
2 cups mushrooms, sliced
2 cups frozen organic spinach
16 ounces organic low-fat cottage cheese
1 teaspoon oregano
1 teaspoon basil
1 jar Newman's Own Sockarooni Sauce
2 cups organic low-fat mozzarella cheese

Preheat the oven to 375°F. In a large pot, cook the lasagna noodles according to the package directions. Rinse, drain, and set the noodles aside.

In a sauté pan, brown the ground turkey over medium heat and add the desired amount of Spike or other all-purpose seasoning.

Drain the turkey and set aside. Add the olive oil to the sauté pan and throw in the mushrooms and spinach. Sauté over medium heat until the vegetables soften.

In a large bowl, mix together the cottage cheese, mushrooms, spinach, oregano, and basil. In a rectangular baking dish, spread a layer of the cottage cheese mixture and top with the browned turkey and Sockarooni Sauce. Add a layer of lasagna noodles on top. Repeat this process. Finish by sprinkling the mozzarella cheese on top. Cover the baking dish with aluminum foil and bake for 25–30 minutes. Remove the foil and bake another 10 minutes so the mozzarella cheese can become golden brown. Allow to cool a few minutes before cutting into squares and serving.

Dr. Crinnion's Favorite Cocktail
(Serves 1)

    ice cubes
    sparkling water
    organic berry juice

Put a few ice cubes into a glass. Pour sparkling water into the glass until it's about three-quarters full. Then add your favorite organic berry juice and stir. This makes a great, alcohol-free evening cocktail.

CHAPTER 9

A Fourteen-Day Menu Plan

Chapter 8 contains a number of wonderful breakfast, lunch, and dinner recipes that incorporate the dietary recommendations found in the earlier chapters. You can create a wide variety of meal plans by selecting different combinations of breakfasts, lunches, and dinners. My wife, Kelly, and I have created the following meal plan in case you want a little more guidance for getting started or you'd like to save time by letting us plan your menus for you.

Meals followed by an asterisk indicate recipes found in chapter 8. The following beverages can be added to the meals.

Drinks
- Water, water, water (drinking 5 to 6 percent of your body weight is a good idea, and lemon or lime slices can really give a delicious fresh boost of flavor).
- Green tea (iced or hot; Starbucks has fabulous antioxidant-rich iced green tea). The addition of a lemon slice helps you absorb more of the beneficial compounds in the green tea.

- Coffee in moderation (1 or 2 cups per day of half regular mixed with half decaffeinated is best to prevent being overcaffeinated).
- Sparkling water (try it with sprigs of fresh mint leaves for a refreshing treat).
- Herbal teas (drink to your heart's content—iced or hot can be delicious).
- Red wine in moderation (one glass per day; organic red wine especially provides incredible antioxidant power).

Day 1

Breakfast

Canadian Bacon, Green Pepper, and Onion Quiche*

Lunch

Healthy Chef Salad*

Snack

Protein Mango Smoothie with Yogurt*

Dinner

Bean and Cheese Soft Tacos with Homemade Salsa*

Day 2

Breakfast

Quinoa, Fruit, and Nut Cereal*

Lunch

Turkey Avocado Wrap*

Snack

Handful of pecans and dried cranberries

Dinner

Baked Salmon over Pesto Pasta*

Day 3

Breakfast

Egg-White Omelet with Mushrooms, Havarti, and Dill*

Lunch

Mozzarella, Tomato, and Pesto on Herb Baguette*

Snack

1 hard-boiled egg with 1 cup organic strawberries

Dinner

Teriyaki Salmon Salad*

Day 4

Breakfast

Gluten-Free Pecan Pancakes, Protein-Style*

Lunch

Chicken Salad with Rice Crackers*

Snack

1 ounce smoked turkey with, 1 slice avocado and 1 organic apricot

Dinner

Baked Tofu with Stir-Fried Vegetables over Brown Rice*

Day 5

Breakfast

Fresh Pineapple, Cottage Cheese, and Almonds*

Lunch

Shrimp Salad Ooh La La!*

Snack

Half of an organic apple with 1 teaspoon organic peanut butter

Dinner

Turkey Sausage and Peppers over Brown Rice*

Day 6

Breakfast

Protein-Style Oatmeal with Nuts and Fruit*

Lunch

Healthy Italian Wedding Soup*

Snack

1 ounce low-fat organic cheese with eight rice crackers

Dinner

Dr. Crinnion's Excellent Chicken and Vegetable Enchiladas*

Day 7

Breakfast

Sunrise Apple Salad and Turkey Bacon*

Lunch

Salmon Spread and Mixed Greens*

Snack

½ cup organic plain low-fat yogurt and ½ cup organic grapes

Dinner

Rosemary Baked Chicken with Orange Rice and Broccoli*

Day 8

Breakfast

Broccoli and Cheese Frittata*

Lunch

Shrimp and Avocado Soup*

Snack

Handful of almonds and dried blueberries

Dinner

Salmon and Vegetable Tacos*

Day 9

Breakfast

Scrambled Eggs, Tofu, and Broccoli*

Lunch

Turkey BLT and Fruit*

Snack

1 cup cubed watermelon with 1 ounce low-fat organic cheese

Dinner

BBQ Chicken with Mashed Butternut Squash and Broccoli Salad*

Day 10

Breakfast

Energy Boosting Smoothie*

Lunch

Easy Turkey Chili*

Snack

2 slices tomato with 1 ounce low-fat organic mozzarella cheese

Dinner

Baked Scallops with Risotto and Artichokes*

Day 11

Breakfast

Nourishing Granola with Milk and Berries*

Lunch

Salmon Salad with Fresh Fruit Salsa*

Snack

1 scoop Amino ICG protein powder shaken with 1 cup soy milk

Dinner

Turkey Burgers BBQ-Style with Sweet Potato Baked Fries*

Day 12

Breakfast

Vegetable Benedict*

Lunch

Grilled Chicken, Cantaloupe, and Pear Salad*

Snack

1 slice gluten-free cinnamon raisin toast with 1 teaspoon organic peanut butter

Dinner

Spaghetti Squash with Ground Turkey Tomato Sauce*

Day 13

Breakfast

Scrambled Egg Whites, Grits, and Turkey Bacon*

Lunch

Tofu and Stir-Fry Vegetable Salad*

Snack

1 ounce lean ham and 1 ounce organic low-fat cheese on a brown rice cake

Dinner

Turkey, Spinach, and Mushroom Lasagna*

Day 14

Breakfast

Vegetable Breakfast Burritos*

Lunch

Chicken Salad on Mixed Greens with Berries*

Snack

¼ cup organic low-fat cottage cheese with 1 organic peach, sliced

Dinner

Teriyaki Noodles, Scallops, and Vegetable Stir-Fry*

CHAPTER 10

Moving Forward

It is my fervent hope that all of my research and clinical partnerships with my patients over the past twenty-seven years will shed light on what may be the real cause of your health problems. Since you are reading this book, you are obviously alive and breathing in air, eating foods, and drinking water, all of which contain a host of toxic chemicals. Typically, on a daily level none of these doses is enough to make you acutely ill, but as they build up over the years, they can begin to rob you of your vibrancy. My patients have shown me the devastating effects of these everyday exposures. Those who have agreed to do the cleansing procedures outlined in this book have shown me the great power of the body to heal itself when its toxin load is reduced. The body's ability to carry an immense burden of toxins—and to bounce back to a healthy state when much of that burden is lifted—continues to amaze me as I work with patients at the Southwest College of Naturopathic Medicine.

What astounds me even more is that this information isn't commonly known. In fact, much of it may be news to your medical doctor and his or her staff, as well as to your dentist, chiropractor, massage therapist, nutritionist, and any other health care provider you work with.

Most of us are aware that our environment is flush with toxins, and cancer is still the illness most associated with toxins. Though certain cancers are clearly linked to exposure to chemicals such as pesticides and solvents, the breadth of toxin-related health problems is so much greater than that. I believe that toxicity testing and the protocols set forth in this book should be the first steps taken for anyone with developing health problems. This goes for all of you who are losing your vitality and thinking you must just be getting old.

It is so unfortunate that the information about the health effects of our everyday exposures is not known to most people. This information is, however, readily available in many medical and scientific journals that can easily be accessed though the government Web site www .ncbi.nlm.nih.gov/sites/entrez?db=pubmed. The best of the journals in this field is also a government-sponsored entity, *Environmental Health Perspectives*. It's available for free online from the Web site www .ehponline.org. So your medical professional can have access to this information, but he or she has to hunt for it because it probably won't be presented at annual conferences or in specialty medical journals. In fact, toxicology specialists still insist there aren't adverse health effects from a buildup of everyday toxic exposures, but only from exposures to levels that would cause an acute poisoning (for example, a pesticide spill or some other industrial or agricultural accident).

These are all reasons that I offer environmental training classes for physicians, and why I wrote this book. Your doctor may not know about toxins, but at least after reading this book you do. It's been said before that knowledge is power, but power that isn't used doesn't do anyone much good. I hope that taking action on the steps outlined in this book doesn't prove overwhelming for you. I've tried to make the steps in the four-week plan small and manageable—power you can use. But don't feel bad if you can't get them all accomplished in thirty days. It may take some people six to twelve months. It doesn't really matter how long it takes you to get these measures into place—it just matters that you do. Because at that point, your body will start becoming less toxic rather than more toxic, and every day that you're moving in that direction is of great benefit to you.

The people who underwent intensive cleansing protocols at my old clinic in Seattle needed that intensive treatment because their health problems were causing so much trouble in their daily lives. As one of my cancer patients told me when he sought my care, "I have one foot in the grave and another on a banana peel." For three months, he devoted about forty hours a week to the intensive cleansing program, and he was rewarded with the disappearance of his primary tumor (which had already withstood maximum radiation and chemotherapy) and metastases to his spine and liver.

The percentage of my patients who have needed cleansing this intensive is low; most have had the luxury of cleansing more slowly. But if you think you need a more intensive program than is mapped out in this book, you can go to my Web site, www.crinnionmedical .com, and look up the list of physicians who have taken my environmental training. I hope that you'll find one fairly close to you who can help support you on such a program. If you don't need that much cleansing care, any of these physicians will be able to help assess your burden of heavy metals, chlorinated pesticides, PCBs, and other toxic compounds.

If you're planning to have children soon, I would urge you to get preconception testing for the toxins that are most likely to cause adverse health problems for your offspring and heartache for you. I've worked with many families whose children had experienced serious health problems that were traced back to the heavy-metal burden that the mother unintentionally passed on to them. These tests are readily available, easy to do, and reasonably priced. The small investment can pay huge dividends in your life and the lives of your family members.

While the available tests cover only a few of the multitude of toxins that may be in your body, they are available for most of the worst toxins. Despite the limitations of these tests, they can give you enough information to know whether you're carrying a heavy toxic load. If you're not, maybe you're one of the lucky ones with great genetics and dietary habits and less severe health problems than many others have. These tests can also give you information about the sources of your toxin exposure. This is invaluable knowledge; without it, you'll continue to be overexposed to toxins on a daily basis. And avoiding continued exposure to toxins is the first step in reducing your toxic load. Like I said, it's best to fix the hole in the bottom of the boat before starting to bail.

To find out whether you're being exposed to heavy metals, it's important that you work with one of the physicians listed on my Web site. While a great number of naturopathic and alternative, or complementary, physicians do heavy-metal testing, not many test for current exposure or know how to spot it in the results. Physicians who have spent the time to study this can spot it, so please utilize their services.

Some sources of toxic exposure can be identified without having to test your blood. A number of foods are known to carry large amounts of toxins in each mouthful. Simply avoid them, starting with nonorganic versions of all of the twelve most toxic fruits and vegetables: peaches, apples, sweet bell peppers (green, yellow, and red), celery, nectarines, strawberries, cherries, pears, imported grapes, spinach, lettuce, and potatoes. Many grocery stores carry organic versions of this dirty dozen, and with a little hunting you should be able to find them. The resources section at the back of this book includes the Web addresses of companies that can ship organic foods to your door. You should also be eating organic meats if you're a meat eater, as well as organic butter and other dairy products. And avoid the fish with the highest mercury levels: shark, swordfish, king mackerel, tuna, orange roughy, marlin, Chilean sea bass, lobster, halibut, snapper, and farmed or Atlantic salmon. These types of salmon are found at restaurants and grocery stores around the country, and, in my opinion, it's the most toxic food you can eat.

Besides avoiding foods known to be toxic, it's also worth getting tested for food sensitivities and allergies. Adverse reactions to foods are a common manifestation of a toxin load that's too high. The most common reactive foods are wheat products, sugar, dairy products, corn, coffee, chocolate, citrus, soy, beef, tomatoes, and alcohol. These can lead to dcbilitating health problems that many people mistake for the normal effects of aging. Ncxt to patients who have undergone cleansing, I've seen the greatest improvements in the health and vitality of people who have been tested for their sensitivity to these foods and then have banned them from their diets.

If any of the above are your favorite foods—foods you eat daily or at least three times a week—it's very likely that you're sensitive to them. The late Dr. Theron Randolph published his work decades ago showing how the consumption of these sensitive foods results first in stimulative symptoms (symptoms that make us feel good) and then move to withdrawal symptoms (allergic reactions, asthma, eczema, arthritis, headaches, fatigue, mood swings, and brain fog). But our brains don't seem to recognize these foods as causing the withdrawal symptoms—our brains still think of them as foods that make them feel better. So when the stimulation wears and the withdrawal symptoms set in, we crave the foods all over again, hoping for a better outcome this time (that is, greater stimulation). In a sense, the cycle becomes an addiction.

On the flip side, it's crucial to know what to eat. From a macro-diet perspective, the standard American diet—a SAD story indeed—is an all-around flop. Much healthier is a diet that's higher in protein and lower in carbohydrates and fats that will cut down on the amount of time that chemicals stay in the body. Several books on these types of diets have been published over the past couple of decades, and for the most part, the diets work very well. Not only do they help reduce cholesterol levels, blood pressure, and overall chemical burden, and lead to weight loss, but they also help women cut their risk of breast cancer and men their risk of prostate cancer.

When we consider foods that increase the excretion of toxic compounds that build up in our bodies, a few emerge as superstars. Number one would have to be dark green vegetables—the deeper the green, the better, since the more chlorophyll we get, the more toxins are cleared from our bodies.

Next on the list are the brassicas (broccoli, cabbage, brussels sprouts, cauliflower, and kale). While the majority of them are green (and kale is deep green) and have a high chlorophyll content, the brassicas also contain other chemicals that help the liver to clear toxic compounds out of the blood. The more brassicas you have in your diet, the lower your risk for cancer and other debilitating diseases (including environmental illnesses) will be.

Another superfood is whole-grain brown rice, which has been the staple of the macrobiotic diet since it was first developed by Michio

Kushi. The fiber content of the grain has been shown to increase the excretion of PCBs and dioxins from both animals and humans. If you don't like to eat brown rice with every meal, you can substitute with capsules or powder. If you include whole-grain brown rice with every meal, you'll be clearing out three times the amount of toxins a day than you would if you consumed it with only one meal a day.

And no discussion of superfoods would be complete without mentioning green tea. Green tea is a heavily studied herb/food in medical literature, and the more studies I read, the more impressed I am. It may be the single most potent health food available. Not only is it a powerful antioxidant, preventing oxidative damage associated with aging, but it protects the brain function, cuts the cancer risk, helps balance the bowel bacteria, and dramatically enhances the ability to excrete highly toxic chemicals.

In addition to making dietary changes, you need to clear the air in your home—and I'm not talking about dark secrets that have everyone walking on eggshells. I'm really talking about eliminating the major sources of indoor air pollution. The Environmental Protection Agency did studies years ago showing that the highest concentrations of chemical air pollutants are inside, not outside, the home. This was true even in towns that were home to chemical and paint plants that spewed millions of pounds of chemicals into the air every year. The indoor pollutants came from smoking in the home, home furnishings (think wall-to-wall carpeting), fragrances, and other chemicals used in the home. Several worksheets are included with the thirty-day plan that can help you make your home a chemical-free (or at least a minimally polluted) oasis. Why not clear the air and let everyone breathe easier? In addition to removing the sources of pollutants, you can buy electric air purifiers (see the resources for more information) and plants that clean the air. In studies done years ago by NASA on plants that can clear toxic chemicals from the air, the top five were:

- Mass cane (*Dracaena fragrans "Massangeana"*)
- Pot mum (*Chrysanthemum morifolium*)
- Gerbera daisy (*Gerbera jamesoni*)
- Striped dracaena (*Dracaena deremensis "Warneckii"*)
- Ficus (*Ficus benjamina*)

If you want these plants to clean your air, you'll need to have a lot of them in any given room. Keep in mind, though, that if you have new wall-to-wall carpeting, neither these plants nor a good electronic filter will keep up with the amount of chemicals being released from the carpet, so it's best to get the carpet removed. I worked with a family who had moved into a new prefab home and within weeks the entire family was ill. I gave them the list of these plants and instructed them to buy lots of them. Within about ten days, all of their symptoms had improved. These plants work very well, but you do have to keep them alive and keep from overwatering them, which can lead to mold buildup.

As you reduce your toxin intake and increase the amount of toxins leaving your body, your toxic load will begin to drop. You probably won't notice anything different for a short time, but as you forge ahead, the symptoms that had insidiously intensified will slowly decrease and disappear. As your toxin load diminishes, your mito-chondrial power plants in each cell will begin to function better, giving you more energy and improved mental clarity. And they'll begin to burn the fat you'd been putting into storage. Certain supplements are also available to help prevent, protect, and optimize your mito-chondrial function. The best are listed in the resources.

These changes aren't meant to be short-term fixes. As I tell my patients over and over, what it takes to get better it takes to stay better. The toxins in our environment aren't going away any time soon, and many of them (the fat-soluble persistent toxins) don't leave our bodies easily without our help. Clearly, as the world around us becomes more and more toxic, we have to continue to protect ourselves with diets and home environments that are as unpolluted as possible. We also have to continue to enhance our toxin clearance and take the supplements that help protect us from these compounds, enhancing their excretion, and protecting the mitochondria. As we continue to minimize our toxic load, our health will continue to improve throughout our lives.

Keeping clean, green, and lean is very much a long-term endeavor, one with your future—and the planet's—in mind. But as for taking that first step, there's no time like the present.

APPENDIX

The Link between Farmed Salmon and Diabetes

Because farmed Atlantic salmon can be considered the major source of the PCBs and other chlorinated compounds linked to increased diabetes risk, doesn't it stand to reason that there would be a correlation between farmed salmon consumption and diabetes rates? Sure enough, the graphs below appear to confirm this.

Diabetic Rate per 1K

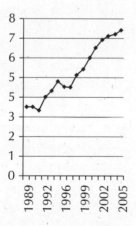

Source: Centers for Disease Control, www.cdc.gov/ diabetes/statistics/incidence/ fig2.htm.

U.S. Farmed Salmon in Metric Tons

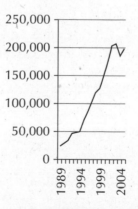

Source: Gunnar Knapp, Cathy A. Roheim, and James L. Anderson. *The Great Salmon Run: Competition between Wild and Farmed Salmon*, TRAFFIC North America, World Wildlife Fund, 123–133.

259

You can see that as the intake of this supposedly heart-healthy meal has risen since the 1980s—when it was reported that eating salmon can help prevent heart disease—the rates of diabetes have followed (the figures represent the number of people in 1,000 diagnosed with it since 1989). Among Americans born in this millennium, one in three can expect to develop diabetes, according to a recent study reported in the *Journal of the American Medical Association.* That's a tremendous increase over the last millennium. While the information revealed in the graphs isn't definitive proof of a connection between farmed salmon and diabetes, it certainly fits with the other information we have about chlorinated compounds and their sources in our environment and this disease. Incidentally, the studies linking salmon and heart disease prevention were conducted with wild salmon, the predominant salmon on the market at the time. The rise of the farmed version came afterward. And these farmed salmon do *not* have even close to the same levels of hearth-healthy oils as the wild salmon do, so their potential health benefit is highly questionable.

1. Reduce Your Toxic Burden and Be Lean for Life

20 *not everyone with a heavy toxic burden* Millikan R, DeVoto E, Duell EJ, et al. Dichlorodiphenyldichloroethene, polychlorinated biphenyls, and breast cancer among African-American and white women in North Carolina. *Canc Epidem Biomark Prev* 2000; 9: 1233–1240.

22 *often leading to early cell death* InSug O, Datar S, Koch CJ, Shapiro IM, Shenker BJ. Mercuric compounds inhibit human monocyte function by inducing apoptosis: Evidence for formation of reactive oxygen species, development of mitochondrial membrane permeability transition and loss of reductive reserve. *Toxicol* 1997; 124: 211–224. Konigsberg M, Lopez-Diazguerro NE, Bucio L, Gutierrez-Ruiz M. Uncoupling effect of mercury chloride on mitochondria isolated from a hepatic cell line. *J Appl Toxicol* 2001; 21: 323–329.

27 *pesticide levels had shot up 388 percent* Hue O, Marcotte J, Berrigan F, et al. Increased plasma levels of toxic pollutants accompanying weight loss induced by hypocaloric diet or by bariatric surgery. *Obes Surg* 2006; 16: 1145–1154.

27 *weight loss and skyrocketing pesticide levels* Chevrier J, Dewailly E, Ayotte P, et al. Body weight loss increases plasma and adipose tissue concentrations of potentially toxic pollutants in obese individuals. *Int J Obes Relat Metab Disord* 2000; 24: 1272–1278.

27 *rose dramatically in their blood* Jandacek R, Anderson N, Liu M, et al. Effects of yo-yo diet, caloric restriction, and Olestra on tissue distribution of hexachlorobenzene. *Am J Physiol Gastrointets Liver Physiol* 2005; 288: G292–299.

28 *Being overweight is a main risk factor* Rylander L, Rignell-Hydbom A, Hagmar L. A cross-sectional study of the association between persistent organochlorine pollutants and diabetes. *Environ Health: A Global Access Science Source* 2005; 4: 28.

28 *refined sugar is free of toxins* Gunderson EL. Dietary intakes of pesticides, selected elements, and other chemicals: FDA Total Diet Study, June 1984–April 1986. *JAOAC Int* 1995; 78 (4): 910–921.

29 *works against the liver's efforts* Anderson KE, Conney AH, Kappas A. Nutrition and oxidative drug metabolism in man: Relative influence of dietary lipids, carbohydrate and protein. *Clin Pharmacol Ther* 1979; 26: 493–501. Leclercq I, Horsmans Y, Desager JP, Pauwels S, Geubel AP. Dietary restriction of energy and sugar results in a reduction in human cytochrome P450 2E1 activity. *Br J Nutr* 1999; 82 (4): 257–262.

29 *Another culprit behind diabetes* Lamson DW, Plaza SW. Mitochondrial factors in the pathogenesis of diabetes: A hypothesis for treatment. *Altern Med Rev* 2002 Apr; 7 (2): 94–111.

2. The Toxin–Fat Connection

34 *of the 413 toxic chemicals being studied* Environmental Working Group. BodyBurden: The pollution in newborns. http://archive.ewg.org/reports/ bodyburden2/.

35 *Obesity rates have more than doubled* Institute of Medicine of the National Academies. Childhood obesity in the United States: Facts and Figures, September 2004 Fact Sheet. www.iom.edu/Object.File/Master/22/606/ FINALfactsandfigures2.pdf.

36 *the EWG tested nine adults* Environmental Working Group. Body- Burden: The pollution in people. http://archive.ewg.org/reports/body burden1/.

41 *meats and dairy products that contained* Tremblay A, Pelletier C, Doucet E, Imbeault P. Thermogenesis and weight loss in obese individuals: A primary association with organochlorine pollution. *Int J Obes Relat Metab Disord* 2004; 28: 936–939.

42 *the less fatty acids were burned* Imbeault P, Tremblay A, Simoneau JA, Joanisse DR. Weight loss–induced rise in plasma pollutant is associated with reduced skeletal muscle oxidative capacity. *Am J Physiol Endocrinol Metab* 2002; 282; E574–579.

42 *deficiencies can prompt people to overeat* Ames B. Delaying aging and optimizing health with diet and supplements. www.zedweb.co.uk/n16health/ aboutus.html#ames.

44 *toxic content can be further reduced* Zohair A. Behavior of some organo- phosphorous and organochlorine pesticides in potatoes during soaking in different solutions. *Food Chem Toxicol* 2001; 39 (7): 751–755.

44 *levels of key pesticides dropped* Lu C, Toepel K, Irish R, et al. Organic diets significantly lower children's dietary exposure to organophosphorous pesticides. *Environ Health Perspect* 2006; 114: 260–263.

46 *In global samplings of butter* Kalantzi OI, Alcock RE, Johnston PA, San- tillo D, Stringer RL, Thomas GO, Jones KC. The global distribution of PCBs and organochlorine pesticides in butter. *Environ Sci Technol* 2001; 35 (6): 1013–1018.

47 *fish is the other top source* Newsome WH, Davies DJ, Sun WF. Residues of polychlorinated biphenyls (PCB) in fatty foods of the Canadian diet. *Food Addit Contam* 1998; 15 (1): 19–29.

47 *A study by the Food Safety Authority of Ireland* Statement from the Food Safety Authority of Ireland Ref: BBC Programme — PCBs in Farmed Salmon. www.fsai.ie/details.aspx?id=7386.

47 *more than seven hundred salmon* Hites RA, Foran JA, Carpenter DO, Hamilton MC, Knuth BA, Schwager SJ. Global assessment of organic con- taminant in farmed salmon. *Science* 2004; 303: 226–229.

47 *children exposed to PCBs while in utero* Jacobson JL, Jacobson SW. Evi- dence for PCBs as neurodevelopmental toxicant in humans. *Neurotoxicol* 1997; 18 (2): 415–424.

48 *Among Lake Michigan fish eaters* Schantz S, Gasior D, Polverejan E, McCaffrey R, Sweeney A, Humphrey H, Gardiner J. Impairments of memory and learning in older adults exposed to polychlorinated biphenyls via consumption of Great Lakes Fish. *Environ Health Perspect* 2001; 109 (6): 605–611.

48 *consumers of high-end fish* Hightower J, Moore D. Mercury levels in high-end consumer of fish. *Environ Health Perspect* 2003; 111: 604–608.

49 *"inadequate data to establish general recognition"* U.S. Food and Drug Administration, "CFR—Code of Federal Regulations Title 21," U.S. Department of Health and Human Services. www.accessdata.fda.gov/scripts/cdrh/cfdocs/cfcfr/CFRSearch.cfm?fr=310.545&SearchTerm=mercury.

49 *Dr. Frederick von Saal recently oversaw a test* Carney, Mike. "Newspaper tests 'microwave safe' labels." *USA Today,* November 17, 2008, http://content.usatoday.com/topics/post/Bisphenol+A/58622204.blog/1.

50 *Microwaving foods in plastic* Castle L, Nichol J, Gilbert J. Migration of polyisobutylene from polyethylene/polyisobutylene films into foods during domestic and microwave oven use. *Food Addit Contam* 1992; 9 (4): 315–330.

50 *disrupters of the hormonal system* Colon I, Caro D, Bourdony CJ, Rosario O. Identification of phthalate esters in the serum of young Puerto Rican girls with premature breast development. *Environ Health Perspect* 2000; 108: 895–900.

50 *higher rates of certain cancers* Marsh, GM. Mortality among workers from a plastics producing plant: A matched case-control study nested in a retrospective cohort study. *J Occup Med* 1983 Mar; 25 (3): 219–230.

50 *BPA's effect on human fat tissue* Hugo ER, Brandebourg TD, Woo JG, Loftus J, et al. Bisphenol A at environmentally relevant doses inhibits adiponectin release from human adipose tissue explants and adipocytes. *Environ Health Perspect* 2008; 116: 1642–1647.

51 *at doses you're being exposed to* Ropero AB, Alonso-Magdalena P, Garcia-Garcia E, Ripoll C, Fuentes E, Nadal A. Bisphenol-A disruption of the endocrine pancreas and blood glucose homeostatis. *Int J Androl* 2008; 31 (2): 194–200.

52 *The higher the mother's toxic level* Smink A, Ribas-Fito N, Garcia R, Torrent M, et al. Exposure to hexachlorobenzene during pregnancy increases the risk of overweight in children aged 6 years. *Acta Paediatr* 2008; 97 (10): 1465–1469.

52 *higher rates of behavior problems* Ribas-Fito N, Torrent M, Carrizo D, Julvez J, et al. Exposure to hexachlorobenzene during pregnancy and children's social behavior at 4 years of age. *Environ Health Perspect* 2007; 115: 447–450.

3. A Different Kind of Diet

65 *chemicals actually become more toxic* Kato R, Chiesara E, Vassanelli P. Factors influencing induction of hepatic microsomal drug-metabolizing enzymes. *Biochem Pharmacol* 1962: 11: 211–220.

65 *toxicity of pesticides, herbicides, and fungicides* Boyd EM, Krupa V. Protein-deficient diet and diuron toxicity. *Agric Food Chem* 1970; 18: 1104–1107.

65 *diets also hurt the immune system* Banerjee BD. The influence of various factors on immune toxicity assessment of pesticide chemicals. *Toxicol Lett* 1999; 107: 21–31.

65   *chemicals remained in their bloodstreams*   Mucklow JC, Caraher MT, Henderson DB, Rawlins MB. The effect of individual dietary constituents on antipyrine clearance in Asian immigrants. *Br J Clin Pharmacol* 1979; 7: 416–417.

66   *diet also helps with estrogen metabolism*   Anderson KE, Kappas A, Conney AH, Bradlow HL, Fishman J. The influence of dietary protein and carbohydrate on the principal oxidative biotransformation of estradiol in normal subjects. *J Clin Endocrinol Metab* 1984; 59: 104–107. Kappas A, Anderson KE, Conney AH, Pantuck EJ, Fishman J, Bradlow HL. Nutrition-endocrine interactions: Induction of reciprocal changes in the theta 4–5 alpha reduction of testosterone and the CP450-dependent oxidation of estradiol by dietary macronutrients in man. *Proc Nat Acad Sci* 1983; 80: 7646–7649.

66   *When measured against blueberries*   Pelligrini N, Serafini M, Colombi B, Del Rio D, Salvatore S, Bianchi M, Brighenti F. Total antioxidant capacity of plant foods, beverages and oils consumed in Italy assessed by three different in vitro assays. *J Nutr* 2003; 133: 2812–2819.

66   *Similar results were found*   Blomhoff R. Antioxidant and oxidative stress. *Tidssker Nor Laegeforen* 2004; 124 (12): 1643–1645. Wang S, Jiao H. Scavenging capacity of berry crops on superoxide radicals, hydrogen peroxide, hydroxyl radicals, and singlet oxygen. *J Agric Food Chem* 2000: 48 (11): 5677–5684.

66   *blackberries' antioxidant strength differs*   Wang SY, Lin HS. Antioxidant activity in fruits and leaves of blackberry, raspberry, and strawberry varies with cultivar and developmental stage. *J Agric Food Chem 2000*; 48 (2): 140–146.

67   *ability to reverse the suppression*   Serraino I, Dugo L, Dugo P, et al. Protective effects of cyaniding-3-0-glucoside from blackberry extract against peroxynitrite-induced endothelial dysfunction and vascular failure. *Life Sci* 2003: 73 (9): 1097–1114.

68   *Drinking green tea on a regular basis*   Setiawan VW, Zhang ZF, Yu GP, Lu QY, Li YL, Lu ML, Wang MR, et al. Protective effect of green tea on the risks of chronic gastritis and stomach cancer. *Int J Cancer* 2001; 600–604.

69   *an even greater reduction in risk*   Zhang M, Binns CW, Lee AH. Tea consumption and ovarian cancer risk: A case-control study in China. *Canc Epidem Biomark Prev* 2002; 11: 713–718.

69   *only one man had developed a tumor*   Bettuzzi S, Brausi M, Rizzi F, Castagnetti G, Peracchia G, Corti A. Chemoprevention of human prostate cancer by oral administration of green tea catechins in volunteers with high-grade prostate intraepithelial neoplasia: A preliminary report from a one-year proof-of-principle study. *Cancer Res* 2006 Jan 15; 66 (2): 1234–1240.

69   *People who drink two or more cups*   Kuriyama S, Hozawa A, Ohmori K, Shimazu T, Matsui T, Ebihara S, Awata S, Nagatomi R, Arai H, Tsuji I. Green tea consumption and cognitive function: A cross-sectional study from the Tsurugaya Project 1. *Am J Clin Nutr* 2006 Feb; 83 (2): 355–361.

70   *they can also chelate iron*   Mandel S, Amit T, Reznichenko L, Weinreb O, Youdin MB. Green tea catechins as brain-permeable, natural iron chelators-antioxidants for the treatment of neurodegenerative disorders. *Mol Nutr Food Res* 2006; 50 (2): 229–234.

70   *green tea blocks the neurotoxin MPTP's ability*   Mandel S, Maor G, Youdim MB. Iron and alpha-synuclein in the substantia nigra of MPTP-treated mice: Effect of neuroprotective drugs R-apomorphine and green tea polyphenol epigallocatechin-3-gallate. *J Mol Neurosci* 2004; 24: 401–416.

70   *shown to have an antianxiety effect*   Vignes M, Maurice T, Lanté F, Nedjar M, Thethi K, Guiramand J, Récasens M. Anxiolytic properties of green tea polyphenol (-)-epigallocatechin gallate (EGCG). *Brain Res* 2006 Sep 19; 1110 (1): 102–115.

70   *about 30 percent less likely to die*   Kuriyama S, Shimazu T, Ohmori K, Kikuchi N, Nakaya N, Nishino Y, Tsubono Y, Tsuji I. Green tea consumption and mortality due to cardiovascular disease, cancer, and all causes in Japan: The Ohsaki study. *JAMA* 2006 Sep 13; 296 (10): 1255–1265.

70   *levels of normal healthy intestinal bacteria*   Goto K, Kanaya S, Nishikawa T, Hara H, Terada A, Ishigami T, Hara Y. The influence of tea catechins on fecal flora of elderly residents in long-term care facilities. *Ann Long-Term Care* 1998; 6: 43–48.

71   *a reduction in the compounds*   Goto K, Kanaya S, Ishigami T, Hara Y. The effects of tea catechins on fecal conditions of elderly residents in a long-term care facility. *J Nutr Sci Vitaminol* 1999; 45: 135–141.

71   *shown to prevent chronic atrophic gastritis*   Shibata K, Moriyama M, Fukushima T, Kaetsu A, Miyaaki M, Une H. Green tea consumption and chronic atrophic gastritis: A cross-sectional study in a green tea production village. *J Epidemiol* 2000; 10 (5): 310–316.

71   *the risk of green tea drinkers developing*   Setiawan VW, Zhang ZF, Yu GP, Lu QY, et al. Protective effect of green tea on the risks of chronic gastritis and stomach cancer. *Int J Cancer* 2001; 92: 600–604.

74   *level of mitochondrial function dropped*   Veerkamp JH, Zevenbergen JL. Effect of dietary fat on total and peroxisomal fatty acid oxidation in rat tissues. *Biochem Biophys Acta* 1986 Aug 14; 878 (1): 102–109.

74   *sugar obstructs components*   Stewart CC, Strother A. Glucose consumption by rats decreases cytochrome P450 enzyme activity by altering hepatic lipids. *Life Sci* 1999; 64 (23): 2163–2172.

74   *A high-sugar diet also impairs*   Peters LP, Teel RW. Effect of high sucrose diet on liver enzyme content and activity and aflatoxin B1-induced mutagenesis. *In Vivo* 2003; 17 (2): 205–210.

74   *volunteers ate a high-carb diet*   Ibid., p. 3.

75   *chemical-clearance abilities recovered*   Leclercq I, Horsmans Y, Desager JP, Pauwels S, Geubel AP. Dietary restriction of energy and sugar results in a reduction in human cytochrome P450 2E1 activity. *Br J Nutr* 1999; 82 (4): 257–262.

4. Out with the Bad

86   *volunteers who consumed 25 grams of olestra*   Moser GA, McLachlan MS. A non-absorbable dietary fat substitute enhances elimination of persistent lipophylic contaminants in humans. *Chemosphere* 1999; 39: 1513–1521.

86   *olestra approach was later incorporated*   Geusau A, Schmaldienst S, Derfler K, Papke O, Abraham K. Severe 2,3,7,8-tetrachlorodibenzo-p-dioxins (TCDD) intoxication: Kinetics and trials to enhance elimination in two patients. *Arch Toxicol* 2002; 76: 316–325.

88   *RBF has been shown to bind easily with PCBs*   Sera N, Morita K, Nagosoe M, et al. Binding effect of polychlorinated compounds and environmental carcinogens on rice bran fiber. *J Nutr Biochem* 2005; 16: 50–58.

88   *dramatically diminishing the reabsorption*   Kimura Y, Nagat Y, Buddington R. Some dietary fibers increase elimination of orally administered polychlorinated biphenyls but not that of retinol in mice. *J Nutr* 2004; 134: 135–142.

88   *wheat bran has shown absolutely no benefit*   De Vos S, De Schrijver R. Polychlorinated biphenyl distribution and fecal excretion in rats fed wheat bran. *Chemosphere* 2005; 61: 374–382.

88   *A study using spinach fiber and RBF*   Morita K, Hamamura K, Iida T. Binding of PCB by several types of dietary fiber in vivo and in vitro. *Fukuoka Igaku Zasshi* 1995; 86: 212–217.

88   *animals eating a diet of 10 percent RBF*   Morita K, Hirakawa H, Matsueda T, et al. Stimulating effect of dietary fiber on fecal excretion of polychlorinated dibenzofurans (PCDF) and polychlorinated dibenzo-p-dioxins (PCDD) in rats. *Fukuoka Igaku Zasshi* 1993; 84: 273–281.

88   *studies of patients with Yusho disease*   Kwon CS, Sohn HY, Kim SH, et al. Anti-obesity effect of dioscorea. *Biosci Biotechnol Biochem* 2003; 67: 1451–1456.

89   *rats fed a diet that was 10 percent nori*   Morita K, Tobiishi K. Increasing effect of nori on the fecal excretion of dioxin by rats. *Biosci Biotechnol Biochem* 2002; 66: 2306–2313.

89   *the group of rats given chlorella*   Morita K, Matsueda T, Iida T, Hasegawa T. Chlorella accelerates dioxin excretion in rats. *J Nutr* 1999; 129: 1731–1736.

89   *lower total body burdens*   Morita K, Ogata M, Hasegawa T. Chlorophyll derived from chlorella inhibits dioxin absorption from the gastrointestinal tract and accelerates dioxin excretion in rats. *Environ Health Perspect* 2001; 109: 289–294.

89   *diet that was 10 percent vegetables*   Morita K, Matsueda T, Iida T. Effect of green vegetables on digestive tract absorption of polychlorinated dibenzo-p-dioxins and polychlorinated dibenzofurans in rats. *Fukuoka Igaku Zasshi* 1999; 90: 171–183.

91   *saponins from plants in the* Dioscorea *genus*   Kwon CS, Sohn HY, Kim SH, et al. Anti-obesity effect of dioscorea. *Biosci Biotechnol Biochem* 2003; 67: 1451–1456.

91   *When tested in mice alongside orlistat*   Han LK, Zheng YN, Yoshikawa M, et al. Anti-obesity effects of chikusetsusaponins isolated from *Panax japonicus* rhizomes. *BMC Complem Altern Med* 2005; 5: 9.

91   *saponins in green tea seeds were able to inhibit lipase*   Han LK, Kimura Y, Kawashima M, et al. Tea saponins and fat absorption. *Int J Obes Relat Metab Disord* 2001; 25: 1459–1464.

91   *a diet including either 4 grams of matcha*   Morita K, Matsueda T, Iida T. Effect of green tea (matcha) on gastrointestinal tract absorption of polychlorinated biphenyls, polychlorinated dibenzofurans and polychlorinated dibenzo-p-dioxins in rats. *Fukuoka Igaku Zasshi* 1997; 88: 162–168.

91   *polyphenol-rich oolong tea*   Hsu TF, Kusumoto A, Abe K, et al. Oolong tea increased fecal fat. *Eur J Clin Nutr* 2006; 60 (11): 1330–1336.

94   *failed to show any increase in glutathione levels*   Witschi A, Reddy S, Stofer B, Lauterburg BH. The systemic availability of oral glutathione. *Eur J Clin Pharmacol* 1992; 43: 667–669.

94   *documented to increase glutathione levels*   Roes EM, Raijmakers MT, Peteres WH, Steegers EA. Effects of oral N-acetylcysteine on plasma homocysteine and whole blood glutathione levels in healthy, non-pregnant

women. *Clin Chem Lab Med* 2002; 40: 496–498. Micke P, Beeh KM, Buhl R. Effects of long-term supplementation with whey proteins on plasma glutathione levels of HIV-infected patients. *Eur J Nutr* 2002; 41: 12–18.

5. Supplements: Your Secret Weapons

103 *short-term vitamin C deficiency* Harris WS, Kottke BA, Subbiah MT. Bile acid metabolism in ascorbic acid-deficient guinea pigs. *Am J Clin Nutr* 1979; 32 (9): 1837–1841.

105 *class of chemicals known as aldehydes* Nosova T, Jousimies-Somer H, Jokelainen K, Heine R, Slaspuro M. Acetaldehyde production and metabolism by human indigenous and probiotic *Lactobacillus* and *Bifidobacterium* strains. *Alcohol Alcoholism* 2000; 35 (6): 561–568.

106 *the highest helpful rating* Gibson PR, Elms ANM, Ruding LA. Perceived treatment efficacy for conventional and alternative therapies reported by persons with multiple chemical sensitivity. *Environ Health Perspect* 2003; 111: 1498–1504.

106 *absorbing the cancer-causing mold toxins* El-Nezami HS, Polychronaki NN, Ma J, Zhu H, et al. Probiotic supplementation reduces a biomarker for increased risk of liver cancer in young men from southern China. *Am J Clin Nutr* 2006; 83 (5): 1199–1203.

106 *green tea extract (GTE) or a placebo* Diepvens K, Kovacs EM, Vogels N, Westerterp-Plantenga MS. Metabolic effects of green tea and of phases of weight loss. *Physiol Behav* 2006; 87: 185–191.

107 *seventy-six overweight men and women* Westerterp-Plantenga M, Lejeune M, Kovacks EM. Body weight loss and weight maintenance in relation to habitual caffeine intake and green tea supplementation. *Obesity Res* 2005; 13: 1195–1204.

107 *significant decrease in their body-fat percentage* Tsi D, Nah AK, Kiso Y, et al. Clinical study on the combined effect of capsaicin, green tea extract, and essence of chicken on body fat content in human subjects. *J Nutr Sci Vitaminol* (Tokyo) 2003; 49: 437–441.

107 *either a capsule of capsaicin or a placebo* Lejeune MP, Kovacs EM, Westerterp-Plantenga MS. Effect of capsaicin on substrate oxidation and weight maintenance after modest body-weight loss in human subjects. *Br J Nutr* 2003; 90: 651–659.

108 *studies conducted in Norway* Takahashi Y, Kushiro M, Shionhara K, Ide T. Dietary conjugated linoleic acid reduces body fat mass and affects gene expression of proteins regulating energy metabolism in mice. *Comp Biochem Physiol B* 2002; 133: 395–404.

108 *all of those who took CLA* Gaullier JM, Halse J, Hoivik HO, et al. Six months supplementation with conjugated linoleic acid induces regional-specific fat mass decreases in overweight and obese. *Br J Nutr* 2007; 97: 550–560.

108 *lost 7 to 9 percent more of their body-fat mass* Gaullier JM, Halse J, Koye K, et al. Conjugated linoleic acid supplementation for 1 year reduces body fat mass in healthy overweight humans. *Am J Clin Nutr* 2004; 79: 1118–25.

108 *CLA group maintained the weight loss* Gaullier JM, Haise J, Hoye K, et al. Supplementation with conjugated linoleic acid for 24 months is well tolerated by and reduces body fat mass in healthy, overweight humans. *J Nutr* 2005; 778–784.

109 *known commonly as rooibos* Marnewick JL, Joubert E, Swart P, et al. Modulation of hepatic drug-metabolizing enzymes and oxidative status by rooibos (*Aspalathus linearis*) and Honeybush (*Cyclopia intermedia*), green and black (*Camellia sinensis*) teas in rats. *J Agric Food Chem* 2003; 51: 8113–8119. Matsuda K, Nishimura Y, Kurata N, et al. Effects of continuous ingestion of herbal teas on intestinal CYP3A in the rat. *J Pharmacol Sci* 2007; 103: 214–221.

109 *a reversal of the state of cirrhosis* Ulicna O, Greksak M, Vancova O, et al. Hepatoprotective effect of rooibos tea (*Aspalathus linearis*) on CCL4-induced liver damage in rats. *Physiol Res* 2003; 52: 461–466.

109 *Rosemary was able to partially prevent* Sotelo-Felix JI, Martinez-Fong D, Muriel P, et al. Evaluation of the effectiveness of *Rosmarinus officinalis* (Lamiaceae) in the alleviation of carbon tetrachloride-induced acute hepatotoxicity in the rat. *J Ethnopharmacol* 2002; 81: 145–151.

109 *boosted the activity of enzymes* Debersac P, Vernevaut MF, Amiot MJ, et al. Effects of a water-soluble extract of rosemary and its purified component rosmarinic acid on xenobiotic-metabolizing enzymes in the rat. *Food Chem Toxicol* 2001; 39: 109–117.

109 *Rosemary has been shown to increase* Zhu BT, Loder DP, Cai MX, et al. Dietary administration of an extract from rosemary leaves enhances the liver microsomal metabolism of endogenous estrogens and decreases their uterotropic action in CD-1 mice. *Carcinogenesis* 1998; 19: 1821–1827.

110 *prevent lung cells from undergoing* Offord EA, Mace K, Fuffieux C, Malnoe A, Pfeifer AM. Rosemary components inhibit benzo[a]pyrene-induced genotoxicity in human bronchial cells. *Carcinogenesis* 1995; 16: 2057–2062.

110 *prevent damage from the very potent toxin* Costa S, Utan A, Speroni E, et al. Carnosic acid from rosemary extracts: A potential chemoprotective agent against aflatoxin B1. An in vitro study. *J Appl Toxicol* 2007; 27: 152–159.

110 *protect brain cells against the toxic effects* Kim SJ, Kim JS, Cho HS, et al. Carnosol, a component of rosemary (*Rosmarinus officinalis* L.) protects nigral dopaminergic neuronal cells. *Neuroreport* 2006; 17: 1729–1733.

112 *a number of powerful liver toxins* Deshpande UR, Gadre SG, Raste AS, et al. Protective effect of turmeric (Curcuma longa) extract on carbon tetrachloride-induced liver damage in rats. *Indian J Exp Biol* 1998; 36: 573–577. Soni KB, Rajan A, Kuttan R. Reversal of aflatoxin induced liver damage by turmeric and curcumin. *Cancer Lett* 1992; 66: 115–121. Vanisree AJ, Sudha N. Curcumin combats against cigarette smoke and ethanol-induced lipid alterations in rat lung and liver. *Mol Cell Biochem* 2006; 288: 115–123.

112 *boost phase 2 enzymes* Goud VK, Polasa K, Krishnaswamy K. Effect of turmeric on xenobiotic metabolizing enzymes. *Plant Foods Hum Nutr* 1993; 44: 87–92. Iqbal M, Sharma SD, Okazaki Y, et al. Dietary supplementation of curcumin enhances antioxidant and phase II metabolizing enzymes in ddY male mice: Possible role in protection against chemical carcinogenesis and toxicity. *Pharmacol Toxicol* 2003; 92: 33–38.

112 *women who took vitamin E* Traber MG, Frei B, Beckman JS. Vitamin E revisited: Do new data validate benefits for chronic disease prevention? *Curr Opin Lipidol* 2008; 19 (1): 30–38.

113 *prevent chemicals from damaging* Sherer TB, Richardson JR, Testa CM, Seo BB, et al. Mechanism of toxicity of pesticides acting at complex 1:

Relevance to environmental etiologies of Parkinson's disease. *J Neurochem* 2007; 100 (6): 1469–1479.

113 *It's also a powerful antioxidant* Eckert A, Keil U, Kressmann S, Schindowski K, et al. Effects of EGb 761 Ginkgo biloba extract on mitochondrial function and oxidative stress. *Pharmacopsych* 2003; 36 (Suppl 1): 515–523.

113 *protects the cells from oxidative damage* Youdim KA, Martin A, Joseph JA. Incorporation of the elderberry anthocyanins by endothelial cells increases protection against oxidative stress. *Free Radic Biol Med* 2000; 29 (1): 51–60.

114 *Elderberry extracts can also curb the oxidation* Abuja PM, Murkovic M, Pfannhauser W. Antioxidant and prooxidant activities of elderberry (*Samucus nigra*) extract in low-density lipoprotein oxidation. *J Agric Food Chem* 1998; 46: 4091–4096.

114 *the production of chemical messengers* Barak V, Halperin T, Kalickman I. The effect of Sambucol, a black elderberry-based, natural product, on the production of human cytokines: I. Inflammatory Cytokines. *Eur cytokine Netw* 2001; 12: 290–296. Barak V, Birkenfeld S, Halperin T, Kalickman I. The effect of herbal remedies on the production of human inflammatory and anti-inflammatory cytokines. *Isr Med Assoc J* 2002; 4: S919–922.

114 *shown the ability to fight colds* Morag AM, Mumcuoglu M, Baybikov T, et al. Inhibition of sensitive and acyclovir-resistant HSV-1 strains by an elderberry extract in vitro. *Z Phytother* 1997; 25: 97–98. Serkedjieva J, Manolova N, Zgorniak-Wowosielska I, et al. Antiviral activity of the infusion (SHS-174) from flowers of *Sambucus nigra* L., aerial parts of *Hypericum perforatum* L., and roots of *Saponaria officinalis* L, against influenza and herpes simplex viruses. *Phytother Res* 1990; 4: 97–100.

114 *capable of lessening the infectivity of HIV* Sahpira-Nahor O, Zakay-Rones Z, Mumcuoglu M. The effects of Sambucol on HIV infection in vitro. *Ann Israel Congress Microbiol*, Feb 6–7, 1995.

114 *and the H1N1 swine flu* Roschek B Jr., Fink RC, McMichael MD, Li D, Alberte RS. Elderberry flavonoids bind to and prevent H1N1 infection in vitro. *Phytochemistry* 2009; 70 (10): 1255–1261.

114 *recovered their health in less than half the time* Zakay-Rones Z, Varsano N, Zlotnik M, et al. Inhibition of several strains of influenza virus in vitro and reduction of symptoms by an elderberry extract (*Sambucus nigra* L.) during an outbreak of influenza B panama. *J Altern Complement Med* 1995; 1: 361–369. Zakay-Rones Z, Thom E, Wollan T, Wadstein J. Randomized study of the efficacy and safety of oral elderberry extract in the treatment of influenza A and B virus infections. *J Int Med Res* 2004; 32 (2): 132–140.

114 *prevents the development of atherosclerosis* Huang LJ, Tian GY, Wang ZF, et al. Studies on the glycoconjugates and glycans from Lycium barbarum L in inhibiting low density lipoprotein (LDL) peroxidation. *Yao Xue Xue Bao* 2001; 36 (2): 108–111.

114 *excellent source of the antioxidant zeaxanthin* Weller P, Breithaupt DE. Identification and quantification of zeaxanthin esters in plants using liquid chromatography-mass spectrometry. *J Agric Food Chem* 2003; 51 (24): 7044–7049. Breithaupt DE, Weller P, Wolters M, Hahn A. Comparison of plasma responses in human subjects after the ingestion of zeaxanthin dipalmitate from wolfberry and non-esterified zeaxanthin using chiral high-performance liquid

chromatography. *Br J. Nutr* 2004; 91 (5): 707–113. Cheng CY, Chung WY, Szeto YT, Benzie IF. Fasting plasma zeaxanthin response to *Fructus barbarum* L. (wolfberry; Kei Tze) in a food-based human supplementation trial. *Br J Nutr* 2005; 93 (1): 123–130.

114 *a reduction in the levels of blood sugar* Luo Q, Cai Y, Yan J, Sun M, Corke H. Hypoglycemic and hypolipidemic effects and antioxidant activity of fruit extracts from *Lycium barbarum*. *Life Sci* 2004; 76 (2): 137–149.

115 *enhanced short-term energy storage* Luo Q, Yan J, Zhang S. Isolation and purification of *Lycium barbarum* polysaccharides and its antifatigue effect. *Wei Sheng Yan Jiu* 2000; 29 (2): 115–117.

115 *the responsiveness of the immune system* Luo Q, Yan J, Zhang S. Effects of pure and crude *Lycium barbarum* polysaccharides on immunopharmacology. *Zhong Yao Cai* 1999; 22 (5): 246–249.

115 *white blood cells responsible for fighting viruses* Du G, Liu L, Fang J. Experimental study on the enhancement of murine splenic lymphocyte proliferation by *Lycium barbarum* glycopeptide. *J Huazhong Univ Sci Technolog Med Sci* 2004; 24 (5): 518–520.

115 *an invader is in their midst* Gan L, Zhang SH, Liu Q, Xu HB. A polysaccharide-protein complex from *Lycium barbarum* upregulates cytokine expression in human peripheral blood mononuclear cells. *Eur J Pharmacol* 2003; 471 (3): 217–222.

115 *shown to head off liver damage* Ha KT, Yoon SJ, Choi DY, et al. Protective effect of Lycium chinense fruit on carbon tetrachloride-induced hepatotoxicity. *J Ethnopharmacol* 2005; 96 (3): 529–535.

115 *comparable to milk thistle* Chin YW, Lim SW, Kim SH, et al. Hepatoprotective pyrrole derivatives of *Lycium chinense* fruits. *Bioorg Med Chem Lett* 2003; 13 (1): 79–81.

115 *reverse the suppression of bone marrow* Hai-yang G, Ping S, Li J, et al. Therapeutic effects of *Lycium barbarum* polysaccharide (LBP) on mitocycin C induced myelosuppressive mice. *J Exp Ther Oncol* 2004; 4 (3): 181–187.

116 *the disease's progress was slowed the most* Shults CW, Oakes D, Kieburtz K, Beal MF, et al. Effects of coenzyme Q10 in early Parkinson disease: Evidence of slowing of the functional decline. *Arch Neurol* 2002; 59 (10): 1541–1550.

116 *eating broccoli can dramatically reduce* Hara M, Hanaoka T, Kobayashi M, et al. Cruciferous vegetables, mushrooms, and gastrointestinal cancer risks in a multicenter, hospital-based case-control study in Japan. *Nutr Cancer* 2003; 46: 138–147. Joseph MA, Moysich KB, Freudenheim JL, Shields PG, et al. Cruciferous vegetables, genetic polymorphisms in glutathione S-transferases M1 and T1, and prostate cancer risk. *Nutr Cancer* 2004; 50: 206–213. Ambrosone CB, McCann SE, Freudenheim JL, et al. Breast cancer risk in premenopausal women is inversely associated with consumption of broccoli, a source of isothiocyanates, but is not modified by GST genotype. *J Nutr* 2004; 134: 1134–1138. Wang LI, Giovannucci EL, Hunter D, et al. Dietary intake of cruciferous vegetables, glutathione s-transferase (GST) polymorphisms and lung cancer risk in a Caucasian population. *Canc Cause Control* 2004; 15: 977–985.

117 *broccoli boosts one of the phase 1 enzymes* Murray S, Lake BD, Gray S, et al. Effect of cruciferous vegetable consumption on heterocyclic aromatic amine metabolism in man. *Carcinogenesis* 2001; 22: 1413–1420.

117   *lends a hand to phase 2 enzymes*   Steinkellner H, Rabot S, Freywald C, et al. Effects of cruciferous vegetables and their constituents on drug metabolizing enzymes involved in the bioactivation of DNA-reactive dietary carcinogens. *Mutat Res* 2001; 285–297, 480–481. Lampe JW, Chen C, Li S, et al. Modulation of human glutathione S-transferases by botanically defined vegetable diets. *Canc Epidem Biomark Prev* 2000; 9: 87–93.

6. Your Home on a Diet

120   *a rash of "sick buildings"*   Rogers SA. Diagnosing the tight building syndrome. *Env Health Persp* 1987; 76: 195–198. Menzies, R, Tamblyn RM, Hanley J, Nunes F, Tamblyn RT. Impact of exposure to multiple contaminants on symptoms of sick building syndrome. *Proc of Indoor Air* 1993; 1 (1): 363–368.

124   *greatest personal exposure to solvents*   Wallace, LA, Pellizzari, ED, Hartwell TD, Sparacino CM, Sheldon LS, Zelon H. Personal exposure, indoor-outdoor relationships, and breath levels of toxic air pollutants measured for 355 persons in New Jersey. EPA 0589. Wallace LA, Pellizzari ED, Hartwell TD, Sparacino CM, Sheldon LS, Zelon H. Personal exposures, outdoor concentrations, and breath levels of toxic air pollutants measured for 425 persons in urban, suburban and rural areas. EPA 0589. Presented at annual meeting of Air Pollution Control Association, June 25, 1984. San Francisco, CA.

126   *levels of trihalomethanes*   Lynberg M, Nuckols JR, Langlois P, et al. Assessing exposure to disinfection by-products in women of reproductive age living in Corpus Christi, Texas, and Cobb County, Georgia: Descriptive results and methods. *Environ Health Perspect* 2001; 109 (6): 597–604.

126   *homes in North Carolina and North Dakota*   Wallace LA, Pellizzari ED, Hartwell TD, Sparacino C, Whitmore R, Sheldon L, Zelon H, Perritt R. The TEAM (total exposure assessment methodology) study: Personal exposures to toxic substances in air, drinking water, and breath of 400 residents in New Jersey, North Carolina, and North Dakota. *Environ Res* 1987; 43 (2): 290–307.

126   *The highest solvent exposures*   Wallace L, Pellizzari E, Hartwell T, Davis V, Michael L. Whitmore R. The influence of personal activities on exposure to volatile organic compounds. *Environ Res* 1989; 50: 37–55.

126   *areas with relatively little agricultural pesticide*   Whitmore RW, Immerman FW, Camann DE, Bond AE, Lewis RG, Schaum JL. Non-occupational exposures to pesticides for residents of two US cities. *Arch Environ Contam Toxicol* 1994; 26: 47–59.

127   *exposing mice to a commercially available freshener*   Anderson RC, Anderson JH. Toxic effects of air freshener emissions. *Arch Environ Health* 1997; 52 (6): 433–441.

128   *a restriction of their breathing*   Anderson RC, Anderson JH. Respiratory toxicity of fabric softener emissions. *J Toxicol and Environ Health Part A* 2000; 60: 121–136.

128   *chemical bases for the scents in perfumes*   Eisenhardt S, Runnebaum B, Bauer K, Gerhard I. Nitromusk compounds in women with gynecological and endocrine dysfunction. *Environ Res Sect A* 2001; 87: 123–130.

134   *newly cleaned clothing was brought*   Thomas KW, Pellizzari ED, Perritt R, Nelson WC. Effect of dry-cleaned clothes on tetrachloroethylene levels in

indoor air, personal air and breath for residents of several New Jersey homes. *J Expo Anal Environ Epidemiol* 1991; 1 (4): 475–490.

134 *Elevated levels of a solvent* Aggazzotti G, Fantuzzi G, Righi E, Predieri G, Gobba FM, Paltrinieri M, Cavalleri A. Occupational and environmental exposure to perchloroethylene in dry cleaners and their family members. *Arch Environ Health* 1994; 49 (6): 487–493.

135 *Neurotoxicity—sometimes fatal—was found* Duehring C. Carpet, EPA stalls and industry hedges while consumers remain at risk. *Informed Consent* 1993; 1 (1): 6–32.

135 *A Partial List of the Chemicals in Carpets* Thrasher J, Broughton A. The Poisoning of Our Homes and Workplaces. Seadora, Inc. Publ. 1989, p. 34.

136 *high emission levels of styrene* Hodgson AT, Wooley JD, Daisey JM. Emissions of volatile organic compounds from new carpets measured in a large-scale environmental chamber. *J Air Waste Manag Assoc* 1993; 43 (3): 316–324.

136 *number of reported symptoms declined* Norback D, Torgen M, Edling C. Volatile organic compounds, respirable dust, and personal factors related to the prevalence and incidence of sick building syndrome in primary schools. *Brit J Indust Med* 1990; 47: 733–741.

136 *carpeting was one of the main culprits* Norback D, Bjornsson E, Janson C, Widstrom J, Boman G. Asthmatic symptoms and volatile organic compounds, formaldehyde, and carbon dioxide in dwellings. *Occup Environ Med* 1995; 52: 388–395.

138 *the incidence of respiratory ailments in children* Jaakkola J, Verkasalo P, Jaakkola N. Plastic wall materials in the home and respiratory health in young children. *Am J Pub Health* 2000; 90 (5): 797–799.

139 *Volatile Organic Compounds Emitted* Ruhl RA, Chang CC, Halpern GM, Gershwin ME. The Sick Building Syndrome II: Assessment and regulation of indoor air quality. *J Asthma* 1993; 30 (4): 297–308.

142 *greater risk of experiencing wheezing* Jarvis D, Chinn S, Luczynska C, Burney P. Association of respiratory symptoms and lung function in young adults with use of domestic gas appliances. *Lancet* 1996; 347: 426–431.

RESOURCES

Health Care and Testing

American Association of Naturopathic Physicians, www.naturopathic.org. Find a licensed naturopathic physician (who graduated from an accredited naturopathic medical school) near you.

Centers for Disease Control and Prevention. Check out the CDC's ongoing project to identify the load of toxins present in the average U.S. resident at www. cdc.gov/exposurereport/. Visit www.cdc.gov/Environmental/ for information on environmental medicine.

Crinnion, Walter, www.crinnionmedical.com. I've been providing extended training in environmental medicine for licensed health care providers since 2001. The training uses a combination of lectures on DVDs (with handouts and exams) for home study and three weekend gatherings. The weekend gatherings provide for question-and-answer time with me and guest lecturers and, most important, time to work on integrating the new information into a practice. Monthly phone conferences are also available, along with an online forum. More information and the names of licensed physicians and health care professionals who have taken my training course in environmental medicine can be found on my Web site. And physicians can access the protocol I use for my patients to ensure that tests are done properly.

Doctor's Data Labs, www.doctorsdata.com. Your physician can order urine and blood tests from Doctor's Data to measure heavy metals in your body. Hair analysis for heavy metal presence is not recommended. It's a valuable tool for measuring methyl mercury overload from fish consumption but can't show mercury burden from dental fillings. It's also not sensitive enough to show other heavy-metal burdens. The urine test is the best method for assessing whether you have a body burden of heavy metals.

Environmental Working Group. Read the body burden study funded by the EWG and check out the toxins present in Bill Moyers and the other participants at http://archive.ewg.org/reports/bodyburden1/. Read the EWG study on toxins present in the cord blood of newborns at http://archive.ewg.org/reports/bodyburden2/.

Metametrix Clinical Laboratory, www.metametrix.com. Blood tests are available to check for the presence of the most common chlorinated pesticides, PCBs, and solvents that can lead to obesity and a number of other health problems. Check with your local naturopathic or alternative medical physician to have the blood taken and the tests interpreted. Your physician can also order urine and blood tests to measure heavy metals in your body, as well as blood tests that will measure your levels of antibodies to foods. While not all food reactions can be identified by measuring antibodies, these tests typically find the majority of foods that are causing your adverse reactions.

Nambudripad's Allergy Elimination Techniques, www.naet.com. Find a licensed practitioner who can help you clear out your food allergies and possibly help clear emotional issues as well.

PollutionWatch, www.pollutionwatch.org. Residents of Canada can enter their postal code to find out what industrial pollutants they're exposed to on a daily basis.

Prime Pacific Health Innovations Corp., www.thecolonet.com. The best home colonic unit—the Colonet JR-4—is available from Prime Pacific. Be sure to mention promo code CGL to receive a discount available only to readers of this book. They can be reached at (800) 223-9374, or (604) 929-7019.

Scorecard: The Pollution Information Site, www.scorecard.org. Enter your zip code and click on Get report. On the next page, click on the top chemicals or the top polluters to find out the top twenty industrial compounds that are polluting the air in your zip code, as well as the most common polluters.

Leta Rose Scott. Leta has been working on medical intuitive and energetic healing with my patients for the past decade. She is in the Seattle area but can work with you wherever you are. She can be reached at (425) 867-1813.

U.S. BioTek Laboratories, www.usbiotek.com. Testing for antibodies to foods is available to your local licensed naturopathic physician or alternative physician.

United States Environmental Protection Agency Web site, www.epa.gov/epahome/commsearch.htm. Enter your zip code and find out what industrial toxins are in your area.

World Center for Emotional Freedom Techniques, www.emofree.com. Learn to clear trauma from your body.

For information on ozone levels in your area, and possibly some other outdoor air pollutants, go to your local county Web site. Most of these can be accessed by typing "www." in front of your county name and ".gov" after it. Then in the search box, type Ozone or Air Pollution. You should eventually be able to find a page that shows the current ozone level in your area.

Where to Get Clean, Green, and Lean Food

Bakery on Main. Gluten-free granola. At health food stores and Whole Foods or on the Web at www.bakeryonmain.com/.

Diamond Organics. Organic foods. www.diamondorganics.com.

Ener-G Foods. Gluten-free foods and recipes. www.ener-g.com/.

Gluten-Free Registry. Find local restaurants with gluten-free menus and read customer reviews. Available for on-the-go searches at gfresistry.mobi. www.glutenfreeregistry.com.

Gluten-Free Restaurant Awareness Program. Find local restaurants with gluten-free menus and read customer reviews. www.glutenfreerestaurants.org/find.php.

Local Harvest. Community-supported agriculture. www.localharvest.org/.

Organic Kingdom. Organic foods. www.organickingdom.com.

Organic Mall. Organic foods. www.organicmall.com.

P. F. Chang's. Excellent gluten-free menu. www.pfchangs.com/.
Picazzo's (in the greater Phoenix area). Gluten-free pizza. www.picazzos.com/.
Safeway. Gluten-free products. www.safeway.com/IFL/Grocery/Home.
Trader Joe's. Gluten-free products. www.traderjoes.com/.
University of Massachusetts Extension: Community Supported Agriculture. www.umassvegetable.org/food_farming_systems/csa/.
Vital Choice. Wild Alaskan salmon is available year-round—canned and frozen—from Vital Choice's Web site. The canned salmon is far superior to what's available at grocery and health food stores. It will cost a couple of dollars more per can, but you'll be happy you spent more. Vital Choice even offers canned salmon that is free of skin and bones. Check out Dr. Crinnion's packages at Vital Choice. It will coincide with the menus in the four-week plan. www .vitalchoice.com/index.cfm.
Vitamin Cottage. Gluten-free products. www.vitamincottage.com/.
Whole Foods. Gluten-free products. www.wholefoodsmarket.com/.

Household Items and Furnishings

Allergy Buyers Club
www.allergybuyersclub.com
A broad range of home products, including air purifiers, bedding, bath products, cleaning products, humidifiers and dehumidifiers, home decor, and steam and vacuum cleaners.

Anderson Laboratories
www.andersonlaboratories.com
Tests for indoor air pollution from indoor building materials. Anderson Laboratories will test carpet samples to see whether the chemicals they contain are neurotoxic.

Blueair Inc.
www.blueair.com
17 N. State St., Ste. 1830
Chicago, IL 60602
Phone: (888) BLUEAIR / (888) 258-3247
Offers air purifier product information, where to purchase, customer service, filter information, clean air resources, and FAQs.

Body and Home Organics
http://bodyandhomeorganics.com
P.O. Box 295
Rhinebeck, NY 12574-0295
Phone: (845) 516-4189
Toll free: (866) 619-6898
Online store with products for face, body, hair, spa, baby, household, pets, gifts, men, and holidays.

Bosch: Green Building Resource Center
www.boschappliances.com/greenbuilding/consumers/index.html
5551 McFadden Ave.

Huntington Beach, CA 92649
Phone: (800) 944-2904
Green resource center for Bosch home appliances. Featured products, rebate
    finder, energy savings calculator, and product catalog ordering.

Calphalon
www.calphalon.com
Stainless steel cookware.

The Carpet and Rug Institute
www.carpet-rug.org
Offers detailed information for both residential and commercial consumers,
    including information on the benefits of carpets and rugs, health and envi-
    ronment, how to select the right carpet or rug, installation tips, cleaning and
    maintenance, and additional resources. Also includes general carpet and rug
    industry information, research and resources, and downloadable fact sheets.

Le Creuset
www.lecreuset.com/en-us
Enamel, stoneware, and stainless steel cookware.

Ecomall
www.ecomall.com
Online resource for searching hundreds of sites that carry green products.

Extremely Green Gardening Co.
www.extremelygreen.com
P.O. Box 2021
Abington, MA 02351
Phone: (781) 878-5397
E-mail: info@extremelygreen.com
Organic gardening supply company. Product buying guides and secure online
    ordering.

Gaiam
www.gaiam.com
833 W. South Boulder Rd.
P.O. Box 3095
Boulder, CO 80307-3095
Phone: (877) 989-6321
Products in a broad range of categories, including home and outdoor, yoga
    and fitness, media library, clothing, and fair trade products. The Web site
    also includes an informational wellness clinic with advice on natural heal-
    ing, whole nutrition, and alternative therapies. Shop online or order a print
    catalog.

Gaiam Life
http://life.gaiam.com
Companion Web site to Gaiam that's dedicated to better living. It provides arti-
    cles, videos, and product recommendations on mind-body fitness, health and

wellness, green living, and personal growth. It also offers discussion boards, blogs, and a newsletter.

Gardener's Supply Company: Green Living
www.gardeners.com/Green-Gifts/GreenGifts_Dept,default,sc.html
128 Intervale Rd.
Burlington, VT 05401
Phone: (888) 833-1412
Products for home, garden, and yard.

Gardens Alive!
www.gardensalive.com
5100 Schenley Pl.
Lawrenceburg, IN 47025
Phone: (513) 354-1482
Online store for organic lawn, soil, and plant care; insect and animal pest control; and weed and disease control products.

General Electric Appliances
www.geappliances.com/products/energy
Information on GE Energy Star appliances.

Great Green Gadgets
http://greatgreengadgets.com/gadgets/
Environmental blog.

Green America
www.coopamerica.org/pubs/realmoney/articles/flooring.cfm
Article on eco-friendly flooring.

Green and More
www.greenandmore.com
Phone: (877) 473-3616
Sister site to Allergy Buyers Club. Online shopping with a wide range of product categories, extensive product reviews, environmental assessments, expert advice, a learning center, and online and telephone customer support.

GreenCulture, Inc.
www.eco-furniture.com
32 Rancho Circle
Lake Forest, CA 92630
Phone: (877) 20-GREEN / (877) 204-7336
Learn about GreenCulture's eco-friendly furniture and buy online. Also, eco-facts and decorating tips and guides for a variety of styles.

GreenFloors
www.greenfloors.com
3170 Draper Dr.
Fairfax, VA 22031
Phone: (703) 352-8300

E-mail: info@greenfloors.com
Learn about and buy environmentally friendly flooring and recycled carpet.

Green-Furniture
www.green-furniture.com
Phone: (877) 534-7147
E-mail: admin@Green-Furniture.com
Browse and buy products, learn about the company, and get more information
   in the learning center.

Green Home Environmental Store
www.greenhome.com
850 24th Ave.
San Francisco, CA 94121
Phone: (877) 282-6400
Extensive information and recommendations on environmentally superior products, going green, and environmentally superior services. Includes online
   store; a "toxipedia" with definitions of environmental terms, news, and articles; and organizational history and information.

Green Living Ideas
http://greenlivingideas.com
2016 Park Vista Ct.
P.O. Box 2466
Santa Rosa, CA 95405
Phone: (877) LIV-GREEN / (877) 548-4733
Broad listing of environmental topics, podcasts, online store, and advertising and
   sponsorship information. For an article on energy-efficient household appli-
   ances, see http://greenlivingideas.com/household-appliances/household-
   appliances-the-new-green-standard-for-energy-efficiency.html. For an article
   on organic yard care for every lawn, see http://greenlivingideas.com/lawn-
   and-yard-care/organic-lawn-care-for-every-green-yard.html.
GreenPan
www.green-pan.com/
GreenPan Europe BVBA
Latem Business Park
Xavier de Cocklaan 68 / 7
9831 Sint-Martens-Latem
Belgium
Phone: +32 9 241 76 50
Environmentally friendly nonstick cookware. The Web site provides detailed
   product information, care-and-use tips, FAQs, testimonials, and a newsroom.
   Information only—product ordering is not available.
Products can be purchased through:
      Amazon: www.amazon.com
      Crate and Barrel: www.crateandbarrel.com
      Home Shopping Network (HSN): http://kitchen-dining.hsn.com
      Target: www.target.com

GreenSource
http://shopgreensource.com
Online store with a vast array of healthy and ecologically responsible products.
   Five percent of net proceeds are donated to green organizations.

Green Works
www.greenworkscleaners.com
Natural cleaners manufactured by the Clorox Co. Information on the products,
   FAQs, and daily green tools and tips.

Happy Hippie
www.happyhippie.com
Eco-shopping directory, discussion forum, Happy Hippie education center, eco-
   business directory and reviews, and barter discussion board.

Institute for Bau-Biologie and Ecology
http://buildingbiology.net/
Information on safe home and office buildings.

HEPA Air Direct
www.hepaairdirect.com
Buy HEPA air filters direct from the manufacturer.

IQAir
www.iqair.com
IQAir North America
10440 Ontiveros Pl.
Santa Fe Springs, CA 90670
Phone: (877) 715-4247
E-mail: info@iqair.com
Information on residential, commercial, institutional, and medical air purification, where to buy products, and customer support and service, including
   downloadable user manuals, filter information, air-quality glossary, and
   success stories.

Jonathan Green Lawn and Garden Products: Organics
www.jonathangreen.com/search.php?category_id=c02bd0226aa93f9bc3649a1a4
   2f6df07&category=organic
Information about Jonathan Green organic lawn and garden products and where
   to buy them.

Let'sGoGreen
http://letsgogreen.biz
Online store with a broad range of eco-friendly products, including paper; water;
   lighting; cleaning products; plastic plates, cups, and utensils; BPA-free bottles; and green home starter kits. The Web site also includes green fundrais-
   ing information, e-mail sign-up, and LetsGoGreen.biz media coverage.

Lodge Cast Iron
www.lodgemfg.com/
Cast-iron cookware.

NaturOli
www.naturoli.com/soapnuts/?gclid=CPrNtobBgJgCFREeDQodLQhJDQ
100% natural laundry detergent.

Planet Green
http://planetgreen.discovery.com/go-green/green-furniture/
Article on making environmentally savvy choices in furniture, including a list of
    where to buy it.

Seventh Generation
www.seventhgeneration.com
60 Lake St.
Burlington, VT 05401
Phone: (802) 658-3773
Environmental and green-living tips, product information, coupons, a newslet-
    ter, and where to buy Seventh Generation products.

Shaklee Distributors: Get Clean
www.shaklee.net/orderhere/getclean/getstarted/index
Information on Shaklee's Get Clean home care program and products and how
    to order.

Simple Green
www.simplegreen.com
15922 Pacific Coast Hwy.
Huntington Beach, CA 92649
Phone: (800) 228-0709
Product information, cleaning tips and solutions, coupons, online store, store
    locator, testimonials, contests, and shows and events.

Personal Care Products and Equipment

All Natural Beauty
www.allnaturalbeauty.us
E-mail: info@anbportal.com
Product information, reading room, recipes, aromatic and herbal glossaries,
    online stores, manufacturer information, and e-newsletter.

Intelligent Nutrients
www.intelligentnutrients.com/
983 E. Hennepin Ave.
Minneapolis, MN 55414
Phone: (800) 311-5635
E-mail: customerservice@intelligentnutrients.com
Buy organic products for hair and skin, as well as aromatherapy products, nutri-
    tional supplements, food products, gifts, and books. Also educational infor-
    mation, links to other organic resources, and a press room.

Juice Beauty
www.juicebeauty.com
Phone: (415) 457-4600

An array of organic skin-care products for both men and women, as well as information on why organic is better, a product solution wizard for making the best product choices, a retail locator, press articles and media clips, and customer testimonials.

NaturOli
www.naturoli.com
9299 Olive Ave.
Olive Business Park
Bldg. 2, Ste. 201
Peoria, AZ 85345
Phone: (877) 654-5433
Online store, detailed product information, testimonials, media coverage, and membership information.

NVEY ECO Organic Makeup
www.econveybeauty.com
611 Madison Ave.
Covington, KY 41011
Phone: (859) 261-7895
Buy NVEY organic makeup online or locate a retail store, explore information about organic ingredients, and learn about the company.

Organic Health and Beauty
www.organichealthandbeauty.com
23801 Calabasas Rd., Ste. 1003A
Calabasas, CA 91302
Phone: (800) 430-3501
Organic food; digestion and detox; healing; and face, body, and hair care products. The Web site also provides smart guides to choosing the right products, articles, and resources, FAQs, and more.

Origins
www.origins.com
Natural cosmetics company that offers makeup, skin and body care, fragrance, hair care, and men's products. They include the Origins Organics line of skin, hair, and body products and a skin-care line from Dr. Andrew Weil. Shop online, at an Origins retail store, or at an Origins makeup counter in most major department stores.

Saffron Rouge
www.saffronrouge.com
3971 Lakeview Corporate Dr.
Edwardsville, IL 62025
Phone: (866) FACE-CARE / (866) 322-3227
Learn about and buy products online, read how the company evaluates products, order free samples, and sign up for the Saffron Rouge newsletter.

Skin Deep Cosmetic Safety Database
www.cosmeticsdatabase.org

From the Environmental Working Group, extremely detailed information on a broad range of skin-care and beauty products and manufacturers. Includes full ingredient lists and safety assessments. Search by product, ingredient, or company. Also provides information on how to take action to promote increased safety in the health and beauty industry, safer shopping tips, FAQs, research information, and updates.

Spirit Beauty Lounge
www.spiritbeautylounge.com
Phone: (888) 409-8889
E-mail: info@spiritbeautylounge.com
Shop for organic beauty products by category or brand, access educational information, and read the blog.

Supplements

Not all supplements are created equal, and if you buy on the basis of price alone, you may end up with the least absorbable products. This is why most naturopathic physicians have their own dispensaries attached to their offices. I learned early in my career that I needed to be sure that I not only determined what supplement the patient needed but also that they got a high-quality product. I believe it's part of my job as a physician to know the quality of the supplement manufacturers and to find the products that work best. Your local health food store stocks a wide range of products, but please buy a higher-cost brand. The major stores, such as Whole Foods, often have personnel in their supplement department who are highly trained. My Web site, www.crinnionmedical.com, has some of the better supplements that I've used successfully for years, and they're available for online purchase. This includes the items I use as part of my protocols.

- Liquid Life. A daily liquid with blackberry, elderberry, wolfberry, mangosteen, broccoli, and green tea. www.mitogenx.com/spiritmed.
- Primary Toxin Shield. Recommended multiple vitamins. www.mitogenx.com/spiritmed.
- Sound Nutrition. Ultra Pure Detox Multi. Available at health food stores.
- Thorne Research's Basic Detox Nutrients. Recommended multiple vitamins. Available through naturopathic and alternative physicians.
- Clean, Green and Lean: Whole Body Detox Kit.

The following products are manufactured and distributed to integrative practitioners by Gaia Herbs Professional Solutions (www.gaiaprofessional.com). They can be purchased separately or as a kit. Check with your local naturopathic physician or check on the crinninomedical.com Web site.

- "Clean" products support elimination of fat-soluble toxins. They contain natural pancreatic lipase inhibitors, including botanical saponins from *Dioscorea, Panax, Camellia sinensis,* and rice-bran fiber.
- "Green" products promote healthy liver and lymph cleansing. They contain all the botanicals listed in chapters 4 and 5 to help your liver clear toxins from the blood more efficiently.
- "Lean" products promote healthy fat metabolism. They contain the best natural agents proven to encourage fat breakdown and weight loss.

Agencies and Organizations

Government Agencies

Agency for Toxic Substances and Disease Registry (ATSDR)
www.atsdr.cdc.gov
Phone: (800) CDC-INFO / (800) 232-4636
E-mail: cdcinfo@cdc.gov
Information on toxic substances, diseases, education and training, emergency
    response, publications and products, special initiatives, toxicological profiles,
    FAQs, health assessments and consultations, case studies, and more.

Household Products Database
http://householdproducts.nlm.nih.gov
E-mail: tehip@teh.nlm.nih.gov
Detailed product information in a variety of categories, including auto, home,
    pest control, landscape and yard, personal care, home maintenance, arts and
    crafts, pet care, and home office. Information is also organized by product
    name, manufacturer, ingredients, and health effects.

The National Institute of Environmental Health Sciences (NIEHS)
www.niehs.nih.gov
P.O. Box 12233
Research Triangle Park, NC 27709-2233
Phone: (919) 541-3345
The NIEHS's monthly *Environmental Health Perspectives* is the best environ-
    mental medicine journal being published. Articles are available for free
    download at www.ehponline.org.

Tox Town
http://toxtown.nlm.nih.gov
Detailed information on numerous toxic chemicals, virtual representations
    of environmental health concerns in several imaginary neighborhoods, an
    A to Z index of disaster and health, and educational and career resources for
    teachers. The entire site is also available in Spanish.

United States Environmental Protection Agency
www.epa.gov
Ariel Rios Building
1200 Pennsylvania Ave. NW
Washington, DC 20460
Phone: (202) 272-0167
A wealth of environmental facts and resources, including basic information on
    environmental education, science, and technology; laws and regulations; as
    well as a newsroom and e-mail update subscriptions.

Other Organizations

Beyond Pesticides
www.beyondpesticides.org
701 E Street SE, Ste. 200
Washington, DC 20003

Phone: (202) 543-5450
E-mail: info@beyondpesticides.org
News blog, alerts and actions, discussion of issues, and information on what to
do in an emergency.

Boston University Superfund Research Program
http://busbrp.org
Community and research resources, projects, news and updates, "Ask the
Researcher," RSS news feeds, and BU SRP publication links.

Center for Health, Environment, and Justice
www.chej.org
P.O. Box 6806
Falls Church, VA 22040-6806
Phone: (703) 237-2249
E-mail: chej@chej.org
Information on toxic substances, community assistance, news, and campaign
information.

Children's Environmental Health Network
www.cehn.org
110 Maryland Avenue NE, Ste. 505
Washington, DC 20002
Phone: (202) 543-4033
E-mail: cehn@cehn.org
News and information, resource guide, training manual, and publications.

The Collaborative on Health and the Environment
www.healthandenvironment.org
c/o Commonweal
P.O. Box 316
Bolinas, CA 94924
E-mail: info@healthandenvironment.org
News and events, working groups, and resources. Includes a toxicant and disease
database.

Columbia Center for Children's Environmental Health
www.ccceh.org
100 Haven Ave. Tower III, Ste. 25F
New York, NY 10032
Phone: (212) 304-7280
E-mail: cccehcolumbia@gmail.com
Press releases and scientific papers, facts about environmental hazards and
health risks, resources, and detailed information for parents and families,
health professionals, community groups, and funders.

Environmental Health News
www.environmentalhealthnews.org
A daily publication providing comprehensive news and information about
environmental health issues.

Environmental Working Group
www.ewg.org
1436 U Street NW, Ste. 100
Washington, DC 20009
Phone: (202) 667-6982
Information about health, toxins, natural resources, a chemical index, blogs,
    and news.

Mount Sinai Children's Environmental Center
www.childenvironment.org
One Gustave L. Levy Pl.
New York, NY 10029-6574
Tel: (212) 241-6500 / (800) 637-4624
Video presentations, current projects, how the center can help you, and how you
    can help the center.

Natural Resources Defense Council
www.nrdc.org
40 W. 20th St.
New York, NY 10011
Phone: (212) 727-2700
News, issues, policy, green living, green business, multimedia, and blogs.

Physicians for Social Responsibility
www.psr.org
1875 Connecticut Avenue NW, Ste. 1012
Washington, DC 20009
Phone: (202) 667-4260
E-mail: psrnatl@psr.org
Information on environment and health, security, PSR chapters, social justice,
    PSR's international work, news and events, publications and resources, rec-
    ommended books, and tools for physicians.

Science and Environmental Health Network
www.sehn.org
3703 Woodland St.
Ames, IA 50014
Phone: (515) 268-0600
E-mail: info@sehn.org
Information about the SEHN's precautionary principle, ecological medicine, law
    for the ecological age, ethical economics, guardianship of future generations,
    public interest research, and environmental news.

A Small Dose Of
www.asmalldoseof.org
Information on numerous types of toxins, their effects on the body, where toxins
    are encountered, regulatory agencies, and resources for additional informa-
    tion. Includes precautionary principle, Web-based toxicology references and

PowerPoint presentations, ethical considerations, the history of toxicology, nanotechnology, and teaching resources.

Toxipedia
www.toxipedia.org
Free toxicological encyclopedia "written by experts and edited for accuracy." Also serves as a resource center for discussion forums, educational materials, and accurate information.

INDEX

acidification of body tissues, 92
airborne toxins, 51–54, 121, 257–258
air ducts, 144, 180
air filters, 140–141, 144, 181–182
air fresheners, 52–53, 127–128
alcohol consumption, 164
Alaskan salmon, 64
aldehydes, 105
alkalinizing urine, 92–93
Alli (orlistat), 90
allopathic medicine, 4
animal fat, 27
anthocyanidin, 66, 68
antibacterial compounds, 131
antioxidants, 66–67, 101–102, 112–116
Apple and Pear Breakfast
    Smoothie, 199
apples, 41, 42, 186–187
aromatic hydrocarbons, 53
arsenic, 53
art of eating
    to battle toxins, 66–71, 256–257
    bread and wheat, 77–78
    case example, 80–83
    clean foods, choosing, 45, 61
    dairy products, 78–79
    description of, 60
    fats, 71–74
    fish, 62–64
    lean protein, 65–66
    organic foods, buying, 61–62
    sugar, 74–77
Asian ginseng, 91
assessing
    emotional toxicity, 154–155

toxic burden, 14–15, 152–153, 254–255
    See also testing
asthma, and carpeting, 136
Atlantic salmon, 47–48, 64, 175, 259–260
ATP (adenosine triphosphate), 22
author, Web site of, 254
auto-immune illnesses, 9–10, 21–22, 58

Baked Salmon over Pesto Pasta,
    228–229
Baked Salmon Salad, 214–215
Baked Scallops with Risotto and
    Artichokes, 229–230
Baked Tofu with Stir-Fried Vegetables
    over Brown Rice, 232–233
BAP (benzo[a]pyrene), 51–52, 53
basil, 196
Bastyr University, 3
BBQ Chicken with Mashed Butternut
    Squash and Broccoli Salad, 234–235
Bean and Cheese Soft Tacos with
    Homemade Salsa, 238–239
beans, cooking, 173–174
behavior, aligning with goals, 101
benzo(a)pyrene (BAP), 51–52, 53
berries, 66–68, 113
beverages, 92, 163, 164, 246–247. See
    also teas
Bifidobacteria bifidus, 105
bioaccumulation of toxins, 35–36, 46
bisphenol A (BPA), 49–51
blackberries, 66, 67, 113
Bliss, Grace, 2, 86
bowel movements, 80, 83–85, 182–184
BPA (bisphenol A), 49–51

bread, and gluten sensitivity, 6–7, 77–78, 167–171
breakfast recipes, 199–212
Breakfast Sandwich to Go, 209
Breakfast Scramble with Sweet Potato Hash Browns, 211
broccoli and brassicas, 68, 96, 116–117, 173, 256
Broccoli and Cheese Frittata, 203–204
brushing skin, 188–189
buckwheat flour, 199
building materials, 121–122, 138–139.
    See also sick building syndrome
Bunless Turkey Burger and Mashed Sweet Potatoes, 213–214
butter, PCBs in, 46

cadmium, 53
caffeine, 107
Canadian Bacon, Green Pepper, and Onion Quiche, 205–206
cancer
    broccoli and, 116
    D-glucarates and, 97–98
    estrogens and, 96–97
    green tea and, 68–69
    personal-care products and, 131
    sugar and, 76
    toxins and, 253
    vitamin C and, 103
Candida albicans, 105
canned foods, 141
capsaicin, 107
carbonated soft drinks, 163
carbon water filters, 142
carpeting, 135–138, 140, 144, 258
castor oil packs, 186
causes, underlying, looking for, 4–8, 31
cayenne, 196
Certified Natural Cosmetics, 133
chelation, oral, 81, 82
Chicken Salad on Mixed Greens with Berries, 225–226
Chicken Salad with Rice Crackers, 222
chlorinated pesticides, 32–34, 39, 42
chlorine filters for showerheads, 143
chloroform, 125
chlorophyll, 88–89, 194
cinnamon, 196

CLA, 108, 196
clean, green, and lean four-week plan
    celebrating, 197
    overview of, 149–151
    setting up, 151–157
    week one, 157–177
    week two, 177–182
    week three, 182–191
    week four, 191–196
clean dozen fruits and vegetables, 45
cleaning products, 143
clearing out toxins
    with bowel movements, 83–85, 182–184
    case example, 80–83
    with chlorophyll, 88–89
    with colon irrigation, 85–86, 184–185
    with olestra, 86–88
    by optimizing liver and kidney function, 92–95, 186–188
    through skin, 188–189
    See also detoxing
clove, 196
coenzyme Q10, 115–116
colon irrigation, 85–86, 184–185
conjugated linoleic acid, 108, 196
constipation, 80, 83–85, 182–184
cooking oils, 73, 151
cookware, 141
cosmetics, 129, 131–134
Cottage Cheese with Peaches and Cantaloupe, 225

D'Adamo, Peter, 3
Daily Greens, 189
daily sources of exposure, 125
dairy products
    avoiding, 6–7, 171–172
    butter, 46
    organic, 62, 176
    as reactive foods, 78–79
dandelion, 110
DDT, exposure to, 32–33
deep cleaning, 180
deep-fried foods, 164
detoxing, 27–28, 44, 118–120, 188–189.
    See also clearing out toxins
D-glucarates, 97–98
diabetes, 28–29, 259–260
diagnosis, keys to accurate, 31

diet
 without detox, 27–28
 fat in, 71–74, 161, 176
 macrobiotic, 256–257
 reactive foods in, 6–7
 vegetarian, 65, 96, 173–174
 yo-yo, 7, 75
dinner recipes, 228–245
dioxins, 54
dirty dozen fruits and vegetables,
  43, 255
dishwashing liquids, 142
DMPS, 82
DMSA, 81, 82
Dr. Crinnion's recipes
 Berry Wonderful Breakfast, 200
 Excellent Chicken and Vegetable
  Enchiladas, 231–232
 Favorite Cocktail, 245
drinks in menu plan. *See* beverages
dry cleaning, 134–135
dry skin brushing, 188–189

Easy Chicken Salad over Greens,
  212–213
Easy Turkey Chili, 219
eating clean and green, 59–60. *See also*
  art of eating; clean, green, and lean
  four-week plan
eggs, organic, 62, 175
Egg-White Omelet with Gluten-
  Free Cinnamon Raisin Toast,
  206–207
Egg-White Omelet with Mushrooms,
  Havarti, and Dill, 210
elderberry, 113–114
electrical cords, 140
elimination diet, 165–167
Ely, John, 103
emotional freedom technique, 155
emotional toxicity, assessing, 154–155
endocrine disrupters, 131
Energy Boosting Smoothie, 210–211
energy-zapping foods, 162–164
environmental medicine, 3–4, 13
environmental training classes, 253, 254
essential fats, 71
estrogens, metabolism of, 95–97
exercise, 8

fabric softeners, 128
farmed salmon, 47–48, 64, 175, 259–260
fast foods, 164
fat
 in diet, 71–74, 161, 176
 inhibiting absorption of, 90–92
 supplements that fight, 106–108
 toxins stored in, 23–25, 27
fatigue, 24
female hormones, 128–129, 131
fiber, 194. *See also* rice bran fibers
fibromyalgia, 24
fish
 actions to take with, 161
 eating, 175, 259–260
 mercury in, 48–49, 62–64, 255
 PCBs in, 47–48
fish oils, 72–73, 195
flaxseed meal, 96
flooring, 144. *See also* carpeting
foam pillows and mattresses, 140
food sensitivities, 6–7, 77–78, 164–172,
  255–256
formaldehyde, 122
fourteen-day menu plan, 246–251
four-week plan. *See* clean, green, and
  lean four-week plan
fragrances, 128–129, 130, 132
free radicals, 66–68, 112
Fresh Pineapple, Cottage Cheese, and
  Almonds, 208
fruit, 43, 45, 172, 173, 255
Fruit and Cottage Cheese, 200
fruit juices, 67, 164
Fruit Salad Topped with Yogurt,
  215–216
Fruit, Yogurt, and Granola, 200
furans, 54
furnace filters, 180
furniture, pressboard, 144

garlic, 196
getting clean
 definition of, 149
 in home environment, 178–180
 from internal toxic load, 182–189
 steps for, 159–172
 supplements for, 191–194
ginkgo biloba, 113, 195

glucuronide pathway, 97–98
glutathione, 94–95, 104
gluten-free recipes
    Apple Cinnamon Pancakes with
      Turkey Bacon, 202–203
    Pecan Pancakes, Protein-Style, 207
    Pizza with Turkey Sausage, Peppers,
      and Mushrooms, 233–234
gluten sensitivity, 6–7, 77–78, 167–171
goals, aligning behavior with, 101
going green
    definition of, 149
    in home environment, 181–182
    from internal toxic load, 189–191
    steps for, 172–177
    supplements for, 194–196
government agencies, role of, 39
green tea, 68–71, 92, 106–107, 190, 196,
    257
green tea extract (GTE), 106–107, 190
green vegetables, 189. *See also* broccoli
    and brassicas
Grilled Chicken, Cantaloupe, and Pear
    Salad, 224

Hard-Boiled Eggs, Fruit Salad, and
    Toast, 207–208
HCB (hexachlorobenzene), 27, 52, 54
Healthy Chef Salad, 221
Healthy Italian Wedding Soup, 218
heavy-metal chelators, 82
heavy-metal testing, 254–255
hepatic recycling, 88
herbs and spices, 101–102, 108–112,
    190–191, 196
hexachlorobenzene (HCB), 27, 52, 54
high-fructose corn syrup, 75, 162
home environment
    air fresheners, 127–128
    building materials, 121–122, 138–139
    carpeting, 135–138, 140, 144, 258
    case example, 118–120
    cosmetics, 129, 131–134
    dry cleaning, 134–135
    plants that clean air in, 257–258
    removing toxins from, and replacing
      with green alternatives, 177–182
    soaps, fragrances, and perfumes,
      128–129, 130

toxicity of, 120–127, 139–146
home-furnishings, 122, 139, 144
Homemade Gluten-Free Carrot and
    Nut Muffins with Yogurt and
    Fruit, 212
honey, 76
hormones, female, 128–129, 131
horse chestnut, 91, 190–191
hydrocarbons, aromatic, 53
hydrochloric acid, 183

illnesses
    auto-immune, 9–10, 21–22, 58
    diabetes, 28–29, 259–260
    toxin-caused, 37–38
    See also cancer
immune system, 65, 105, 114, 115. *See
    also* illnesses, auto-immune
immunoglobulin G food-sensitivity
    blood tests, 166, 172
indole-3-carbinols, 116
indoor air pollutants, 121
industrial chemicals, 33–34
inflammation, and fats, 72
insect control, 145. *See also* pesticides
intensive cleansing protocols, 254
intentions, setting, 151–152
interior furnishings, 122, 139, 144
Irish Oatmeal with Fruit and Nuts, 201
Island Smoothie, 199

Jammin' Jambalaya, 237–238

kidneys, 92–93, 186–188

Lactobacillus adicophilus, 105, 106
laundry, washing and drying, 144
L-carnitine, 115–116
lead, 81, 137
leapfrogging phenomenon, 46
licorice, 98
lipase, 90
lipolysis, 26, 52
Liquid Life, 189, 195
liver
    diseases of, 75
    estrogen metabolism and, 95–97
    foods good for, 186–188
    glucuronide pathway and, 97–98

optimizing function of, 93–95,
 108–112, 186–188
 vitamin C and, 103
Liver Cleanse (Thorne Research), 185
local foods, 62
lunch recipes, 212–228
lymphatic system, 188

macrobiotic diet, 256–257
magnesium, 84, 183, 194
mattresses, foam, 140
MEA/DEA/TEA, 131
meats, 62, 174–175
Mediterranean Salad with Grilled
 Chicken, 216–217
menopause, 81, 95
menu plan, 246–251
mercury, 22, 48–49, 62–64, 255
methylation pathway, 97
microwaving foods, 49–51
milk thistle, 98, 110–111
minerals to optimize liver function,
 93–94
Mitchell, Bill, 3
mitochondria
 antioxidants and, 112
 blackberry juice and, 67
 description of, 11, 22
 functioning of, 23
 trans fats and, 74
mold, 143, 145, 180
Mozzarella, Tomato, and Pesto on Herb
 Baguette, 217–218
multiple chemical sensitivity, 10, 58–59,
 105–106
multivitamins, 102, 193
Mushroom, Eggplant, and Swiss Chard
 Lasagna, 236–237
Mushroom, Spinach, and Cheese
 Omelet with Whole-Grain Gluten-
 Free Toast, 203
musk xylene and musk ketone, 128–129

NAC (N-acetyl-L-cysteine), 82, 94–95,
 195
National Research Council, 5–6
natural certifications, 133
natural foods, power of, 2
natural gas appliances, 142–143

naturopathic medicine, 2–3, 4, 10, 12
newborns, toxins passed to, 34–35,
 52, 53
New Orleans-Style Sausage, Beans, and
 Rice, 225
nonoccupational pesticide exposure
 study, 126–127
Nourishing Granola with Milk and
 Berries, 210
nutmeg, 196

obesity, and toxic burden, 6, 19–22
oils, 72–73, 151, 195
olestra, 86–88
olive oil, 73
1,4-dioxane, 132–133
oral chelation, 81, 82
organic certifications, 133–134
organic foods, 40, 41–45, 61–62, 157,
 158, 255
organophosphate pesticides, 41, 54
orlistat (Alli), 90–91
Ornish, Dean, 8
overnutrition, 21
oxidative damage, 67, 112

packaging, symbols on, 133–134
parabens, 129, 131–132
parkinsonism, 70, 110, 116
Pauling, Linus, 103
PCBs (polychlorinated biphenyls),
 45–48, 87–88
peanut butter, contaminated, 110
Peanut Butter and Jelly with
 Watermelon and Apricot Salad,
 226–227
perfluorocarbons (PFCs), 54
perfumes, 128–129, 130
peroxynitrites, 67–68
persistent organic pollutants, 26, 27,
 28, 36
personal-care products, 129, 131–134,
 143
pesticides
 alternatives to, 145
 chlorinated, 32–34, 39, 42
 nonoccupational exposure to,
 126–127
 organophosphate, 41, 54

petrochemicals, 132
PFCs (perfluorocarbons), 54
physical health, rating, 152–153
pillows, foam, 140
Pizzorno, Joe, 3
plants that clean air, 257–258
plastic, 49–51, 138, 141–142
polychlorinated biphenyls (PCBs), 45–48, 87–88
polymers, synthetic, 132
polyphenols, 66, 68, 70, 91–92
pregnancy, 35, 47, 254. *See also* newborns, toxins passed to
probiotics, 70, 98, 105–106, 184, 194–195
produce, 41–45, 62, 160. *See also* fruit; vegetables
protein, 65–66, 173–177. *See also* meats
Protein Mango Smoothie with Yogurt, 208
Protein-Style Oatmeal with Nuts and Fruit, 209
psyllium, 194

Quinoa, Fruit, and Nut Cereal, 201

rancid oils, 73
Randolph, Theron, 256
reactive foods, 6–7
recipes
    for breakfasts, 199–212
    for dinners, 228–245
    for lunches, 212–228
recommended daily allowance (RDA) of nutrients, 102, 192
replacements for favorite foods, finding, 177
research on toxins, 39–40
rice bran fibers, 88, 189, 194
rice pasta, 79
rice, whole-grain brown, 189, 256–257
rooibos, 109
rosemary, 96, 109–110
Rosemary Baked Chicken with Orange Rice and Broccoli, 231

salmon, 47–48, 64, 175, 259–260
Salmon and Spinach over Pasta, 235–236
Salmon and Vegetable Tacos, 236

Salmon Salad, 223
Salmon Salad with Fresh Fruit Salsa, 227–228
Salmon Spread and Mixed Greens, 214
Salmon with Lemon Butter Sauce and Sautéed Zucchini and Yellow Squash, 239
saponins, 91
saunas, low-temperature, 188–189
Scallops with Asparagus and Brown Rice, 243–244
scientific method, 39
Scrambled Eggs, Tofu, and Broccoli, 204–205
Scrambled Egg Whites, Grits, and Turkey Bacon, 211–212
Scrambled Eggs with Gluten-Free Toast and Fruit, 202
Scrumptious Egg Salad Sandwich with Fruit, 220–221
Seared Ham, Steamed Carrots, and Broccoli Slaw, 241–242
seaweeds, 89–90
setting up clean, green, and lean four-week plan, 151–157
shoes, removing, 144, 178
showerhead, filters for, 143
Shrimp and Avocado Soup, 217
Shrimp Salad Ooh La La!, 226
sick building syndrome, 120, 135, 136
silymarin, 110–111
skin, detoxing through, 188–189
smoking, 53, 103, 122
soaps, 128–129, 130
solvent exposure, 52–53, 123
soy products, 96, 174
Spaghetti Squash with Ground Turkey Tomato Sauce, 240
sparkling water, 92
spices. *See* herbs and spices
spinach, 89–90
standard American diet, 65–66, 256
sugar, 6–7, 28–29, 74–77, 162–163
sulfates, 97, 132
sulforaphanes, 116
Sunrise Apple Salad and Turkey Bacon, 208–209
supplements
    antioxidants, 101–102, 112–116

case example, 99–100
for getting clean, 191–194
for going green, 194–196
herbs and spices, 108–112, 190–191, 196
probiotics, 70, 98, 105–106, 184, 195–196
recommended program for, 101–102
uses of, 100–101
vitamin C, 102–104, 193
whey protein powder, 95, 104–105, 194
support team, 155–157, 197
symptoms of toxicity, assessing, 15, 152–153
synthetic colors and fragrances, 132

teas
for alkalinizing urine, 92
green, 68–71, 92, 106–107, 190, 196, 257
for inhibiting fat absorption, 91–92
white, 106
Teflon chemicals, 52
Teriyaki Noodles, Scallops, and Vegetable Stir-Fry, 242–243
Teriyaki Salmon Salad, 228
testing for toxins, 166, 172, 254–255
thermogenesis, 23, 42
Thorne's Buffered C Powder, 166
thyme, 196
tofu, 174
Tofu and Stir-Fry Vegetable Salad, 223–224
Tofu BBQ Sandwiches with Vegetables, 222
Tofu Veggie Wrap, 220
Total Exposure Assessment Methodology study, 124, 126
toxic burden
assessing, 14–15, 152–153, 254–255
changes from reduction in, 258
healing from, 252
toxins
airborne, 51–54, 121, 257–258
avoiding exposure to, 255
bioaccumulation of, 35–36, 46
classes of, 37
effects of, 4–6

emotional, energetic, and spiritual, 14
gradual buildup of, 12–13
in home environment, 139–146
increasing excretion of, 66–71, 256–257
obesity and, 19–22
passed from mothers to newborns, 34–35, 52, 53
research on, 39–40
results after decrease in levels of, 10–11
as stored in fat, 23–25
See also clearing out toxins; detoxing
trans fats, 74, 161
trashing toxic food, 159–161
Turkey and Artichoke Casserole, 238
Turkey and Avocado Sandwich with Grapes, 224
Turkey Avocado Wrap, 219
Turkey BLT and Fruit, 216
Turkey Burgers BBQ-Style with Sweet Potato Baked Fries, 241
Turkey Sausage and Peppers over Brown Rice, 230
Turkey, Spinach, and Mushroom Lasagna, 244–245
turmeric, 112

ureas, 132
urine, alkalinizing, 92–93
USDA Organic seal, 133

vacuum cleaners, 144
vegetables, 43, 45, 172–173, 189, 255. See also broccoli and brassicas
vegetarian diet, 65, 96, 173–174
Veggie Benedict, 205
Veggie Breakfast Burritos, 204
ventilation, 142, 143
Vinaigrette Chicken with Broccoli, 240
vital statistics, 153–154
vitamin C, 102–104, 193
vitamin E, 112–113, 195
vitamins to optimize liver function, 93–94
volatile organic compounds, 139

waterbeds, 140
water filters, 142

water, sparkling, 92
weeds, killing, 145. *See also* pesticides
weight loss
    accelerating, 195–196
    case examples, 19–20, 30–32, 57–59
    clean, green, and lean four-week plan
        and, 149–151
    conjugated linoleic acid and, 108
    as doubled-edged sword, 25–28
    green tea and, 107
    saboteurs of, uncovering, 164–172
    supplements for, 194–195
wet cleaning of clothing, 178

wheat and gluten sensitivity, 6–7, 77–78,
    167–171
wheat flour substitutions, 198–199
whey protein powder, 95, 104–105, 194
white tea, 106
whole grains, 176–177
Wild Alaskan Salmon in Fruit Sauce
    with Brown Rice and Broccoli, 243
wild rose, 91
wild yam, 91
wolfberry, 114–115

yo-yo dieting, 7, 75